# Testimonials

"Amy Riley exemplifies, from authentic experience, how to love the pregnant you while discovering your *unique* way to be pregnant. Recognizing that each pregnancy is different, she empowers a woman to be present in each experience and to explore, create, and believe in her *best pregnant self*, consciously and intentionally making informed choices - accepting the stories of others, yet honoring her own."

– DEBORAH MEGGITT, Pregnancy Coach, Doula, and Prenatal Yoga Instructor

"Amy has lovingly and powerfully created a wonderful tool to support any pregnant woman to go through pregnancy with her eyes wide open and her heart filled with appreciation."

– MELISSA G WILSON, book publisher, marketer, coach, and fifteen-time author

"Bravo to Amy Riley and *Loving the Pregnant You* for shining a necessary light on the concept that our pregnant bodies are to be loved, cherished, and taken care of, inside and out. This book is the perfect companion for real moms-to-be everywhere!

– BETH ALDRICH, Nutrition Education Trainer, Culinarian
and author of *Real Moms Love to Eat*

"Amy L. Riley writes with compassion and clarity for pregnant mothers. This book would be a welcomed, nourishing treat to mark a pregnancy. Amy's words will ignite inner wisdom in every expectant mother who reads them. The reflective questions and anecdotes bring the reader in for experiences to harness memories and self-care in pregnancy. Get this book for your favorite expectant mother!"

– JILL WODNICK, birth doula and creator of
*Prenatal Peace & Calming*™ audio relaxation cd

"In *Loving the Pregnant You*, author Amy L. Riley has explored the many and varied experiences and feelings one goes through during pregnancy. In an open, accepting, and non-judgmental way, Amy provides thought-provoking options for experiencing your pregnancy, your way, while feeling really good about your choices. While I am happy with the many choices I made during my pregnancy, I wish this book was around when I started my pregnancy journey. The many options Amy offers through women's journeys shared in the book would have opened my mind and heart even more to the beautiful possibilities that exist to create your ideal pregnancy."

– JILL HOPE, Founder of *I Shine*

# Loving the Pregnant You

# Loving the Pregnant You
## A Guide to Creating a Life Your Way

By Amy L. Riley, MSTD

ISBN 978-1482318890

www.lovingthepregnantyou.com

# Loving
## the
# Pregnant You

A Guide
to Creating a
Life *Your*
Way

*Pat —
LOVE what you
do for moms & families
& babies! Thank you,
Amy L Riley*

Amy L. Riley, MSTD

# Table of Contents

# Acknowledgements

Kevin – my husband. Thank you Honey, for your support and for listening to my ever-changing, always intense stream of thoughts and feelings. Not only did you listen and work hard to understand me, you got creative and found ways to best support me and our family. You are terrific. I wouldn't want to take this journey with anyone else. You are my perfect partner.

My Mom. Thanks Mom for waiting all this time for me to "get" what-it's like to be a mom – to do whatever you need to for another human being and to just want with every fiber of your being for your child to be happy. And, for waiting so patiently (i.e., not asking or hinting about when it's going to happen) for your eldest child to get around to having kids. I love you Mom.

Lisa – my sister. I looked to you, Lisa, in your first pregnancy to help me determine how I was going to handle all this. I figured that we were sisters, we have some of the same genes, and if you could do this then there was a chance that I could as well. It turns out that you were the perfect person to be watching! You were calm, rational, busting paradigms by running in your third trimester, and made it look easy. I love you.

Mary Jo – my life coach. You were the perfect coach for me when I was contemplating what, at the time, seemed like a nearly impossible endeavor: being an entrepreneur, a good wife, AND a mom simultaneously! Thank you for guiding me to identify and deconstruct the disempowering perspectives I had. You changed my life.

Alison – my writing coach. This book would not yet be written if it wasn't for your constant support and coaching. I can't express enough what it means to me to know that I have your loving and brilliant cheerleading, whenever I need it. Thank you SO much for it. I'd have been lost without it.

Barbara – my editor. Whew, what a journey! Thank you for being my partner throughout and for working with me in the ways that best suited me. I needed your frequent editing comments and feedback (as you well know!). This book would've had WAY too many tangents, unclear points, changes in "voice," and other problems if it weren't for you! You're very good at what you do. And, I loved every minute we got to spend working on it together.

Ellen, Laura, Shannon, Jenny, and all the Tiara Coaching community. Thank you for supporting me and believing that I had something worthwhile to share. Your coaching, your accountability, and your company were invaluable on a day-to-day basis. You brought me back to an "empowering" mindset when doubts or overwhelm crept in and, you kept me writing. Thank you!

# Introduction

Welcome to "Loving the Pregnant You"! I'm glad you're here. And, I want to acknowledge you for being interested in loving yourself while you're expecting. It's extremely easy as humans – and I think especially as women – to expect so much (too much) and to be demanding and unforgiving with ourselves. It is my intent that this book provides you with inspiration and ideas for enjoying yourself and your pregnancy as much as possible.

## Why I wrote "Loving the Pregnant You"

I wrote this book because I wish there had been one like it at the time that I was newly pregnant, and maybe even before I was pregnant. Back when my husband and I were deciding if and when to have kids, I was highly reluctant and cynical about my ability to "do pregnancy well."

The obvious lack of control, the hormone fluctuations, and the responsibility for a little being inside of me – none of this seemed good. I didn't want to gain weight and have my shape change. I didn't want hormones making me feel irritable. I didn't want to be viewed as the crazy pregnant lady. Women's ankles swell, their shoe sizes can change, and they can get special diseases while they're pregnant. I felt I had hard evidence about why pregnancy was a bad deal. Pregnancy seemed like it'd be full of pressure and restrictions. So, as you can clearly see, I had a wholly uninspiring outlook!

With these thoughts and feelings prevalent within me and because my husband and I wanted to have a couple children, I realized I was setting myself up to live years of my life with a "just get through it" mentality. I was looking at pregnancy as something to tolerate, assuming I could never "do" it well. I realized I was creating a situation in which I would not be at my best, that I would simply be trying to "grin and bear it." And, when I saw what I was doing, I realized that I was not committed to living that way! Instead, I wanted to figure out how to love the experience, regardless of what the experience might be. I wanted to give myself a shot at liking myself and what was happening during pregnancy.

At the time, I had been an individual coach with a number of years experience, specializing in working with entrepreneurs. I had been telling my clients they could create anything they wanted for their businesses and their lives. I'd seen people completely shift their perspective from one of resignation to one of inspiration and success. I'd seen areas of my own life transform. So, I knew it was *possible* to move away from my cynical view about pregnancy. Yet, I had no idea *how*.

The shift I eventually created started with belief and commitment. I *believed* it was possible to change my thoughts and thrive during pregnancy. Again, I didn't know how, yet it was enough to believe it was even in the realm of possibility. And, I made a simple *commitment* to myself: I was going to enjoy my pregnancy as much as I could.

And...I did. I enjoyed being pregnant and, more importantly, I loved who I was when I was pregnant. This was my own personal miracle. This was something that previously had seemed completely impossible.

How did I do it? In many different ways. Sometimes it seemed like I was experiencing huge, life-altering insights. And, the vast majority of the time, I was creating tiny little changes for myself that eventually added up to something big.

I was on the constant lookout for my automatic, cynical views about pregnancy and about myself as a pregnant person. When I saw one, I looked at how I could improve it – even by just a little bit. I distinctly remember expecting to feel bad physically during my first trimester. I kept waiting for the morning sickness and indigestion. When someone asked me, "How are you feeling?" I heard, "How badly are you feeling?" I caught myself making the automatic negative assumption and reminded myself that I didn't have to expect to feel bad. I could assume that I was going to feel great.

Our expectations and assumptions can be empowering or negative. When we take on an empowering belief, we often find ourselves taking actions that will help the belief become reality. When I started expecting to feel well, I found myself making sure that I got adequate sleep and continuing to eat healthily. When I had expected my physical well-being to be on a downward slide, I wasn't as motivated to make healthy choices. Because what would've been the point? I was just going to get morning sickness anyway. When I shifted my expectations to more positive ones, I then took actions that supported me in achieving the outcomes I wanted.

I have many examples of when I caught myself expecting something less than ideal. And, I'd ask myself, "Why can't I have exactly what I want? If I assumed I could have exactly what I wanted, what would I do to get it?" It sometimes seemed like a futile inquiry (as my cynical views were still winning out), yet a harmless one. What could go wrong? I was already cynical. So, trying to poke holes in my cynical perspectives could only help. I pretty consistently noticed negative thinking and worked to shift my thoughts.

A huge ah-ha moment occurred for me when I was talking to my life coach (who I purposely hired because she was a mom and an independent business owner) and trying to determine how to work my next tropical-destination vacation around my hopefully soon-to-come pregnancy. I didn't want to "waste" my vacation time while I was pregnant because I wouldn't be able to drink margaritas, I might be fat, I might be sluggish, etc. My coach asked me, "Do you want to be pregnant sitting in your house in Chicago in the winter or do you want to be pregnant strolling the beaches of Mexico?" Ah ha! I want the latter. Why had I not seen that? This was a huge insight for me. I wanted to continue to lead the kind of life that I had created for myself, with entrepreneurship and flexibility in my days, and frequent vacations. And, I could continue to do that while I was pregnant. I could be "me" during my pregnancy. I could continue to live life "my" way. I didn't have to carve out nine months in which I'd downscale or pause my life. It was a huge, empowering mindset shift for me.

At the same time that I was working to shift my thoughts to more positive ones, I didn't try to pretend that I wasn't frustrated, disappointed, ashamed, or feeling other negative emotions at times. For example, when I first started to share with people that I was pregnant with my first baby, people were over-the-top excited for us. My husband and I had been married for a while, and others weren't sure whether we were going to become parents. They were so excited to find out that we were! And, I was ashamed and confused because I wasn't nearly as excited as they were. My excitement was dimmed by my feelings of anxiety and overwhelm. I noticed my reaction to others' enthusiasm, and I did my best to let my negative emotions be. I knew that there was always something to be learned from our feelings and that all our feelings are valid. I didn't try to talk myself out of my shame and confusion. Instead, I saw that my emotions made perfect sense. And so did the emotions of my loved ones. Of course they were excited. And, of course I was anxious and overwhelmed. Deciding to have a baby was a big responsibility. I didn't want to take it lightly. I viewed my feelings as a good sign – a sign that I was fully cognizant of my actions and the consequences.

I chose not to feel bad about myself because I felt some "negative" emotions. I could feel confused and uncomfortable, yet not have to judge myself as a "bad" person or mom. And, I realized that even though I experienced "negative" thoughts or emotions during my journey, it didn't mean that I had to declare the whole pregnancy "negative." I could have both. I could have a range of feelings. I could have unwanted emotions and reactions inside of what I considered to be a wonderful experience! Allowing myself to fully feel and learn from my negative feelings and concerns – without having to write off the whole experience as "bad" – was a highly valuable endeavor.

I tapped into other moms for ideas and inspiration. I asked them about *what* worked for them and about *how* they determined what worked best for them. And, I reminded myself that I didn't have to make the same choices they did. As I listened to other women tell their pregnancy and childbirth stories, I got ideas about possible ways to approach situations, and I realized there was an infinite number of ways to "do" pregnancy. I thought about choices such as how I wanted to memorialize my pregnancy (without pressuring myself to create an elaborate scrapbook) and how open I was to inducing labor past my due date – questions that I wouldn't have considered so intentionally if I hadn't been listening to others' accounts of similar inquiries.

When I heard about significant challenges women faced, I felt inspired by how they stepped up physically and mentally, and I was reminded to appreciate every aspect that was flowing easily for me. I identified what mindsets and actions I thought would work best for me in the face of difficulties. By understanding the kind of pregnant women others were, I discovered more about the pregnant woman I wanted to be.

I saw more and more clearly that I could discover the best ways for *me* to be pregnant. I didn't have to make the same choices that my female friends and family members had made. I could, if the choices made sense to me, or I could go in search of what would best suit me. I continued to strengthen my belief that I could create my unique experience, that I could be pregnant in *my* way.

With a personal commitment and the willingness to tune into and learn from your thoughts and feelings, you can uncover what works best for you and create a pregnancy in which you'll love the pregnant you.

## What I want for my readers...

What I want for the readers of *Loving the Pregnant You* first and foremost is for each of you to love the pregnant you, to like who you are and how you're approaching your unique pregnancy journey. You won't enjoy all moments or everything about being pregnant, certainly. Yet, with a conscious intention to discover the circumstances in which you are your best pregnant self, you can create a great deal of enjoyment and pride.

By telling the stories of many women with very different personalities, perspectives, sets of circumstances, and approaches, this book is designed to provide you with ideas and inspiration that resonate for you. I've interviewed over one hundred women about how they made choices that worked for them, how they dealt with challenges in an empowering way, and how they stayed present to the miracle that baby-making is! Not all the stories will be helpful for you, although some will likely show you exactly what you *don't* want because you'll be clear that what worked for one woman certainly *will not* work for you! And, hopefully you'll run across approaches and perspectives that will create excitement and/or relief for you and will feel wholly empowering.

The opportunity to thoughtfully and intentionally make choices, to not be on autopilot, and to set yourself up to be the pregnant woman you most want to be is an exciting one. I want you – whether you are pregnant, in the process of getting pregnant, or think you might want to be pregnant someday – to be able to be a fly on the wall of other people's pregnancies. And, without any advice-giving, read about the choices that others have made and learn how different choices worked out for women, so that you can confidently and proactively make pregnancy a time to thrive, not a time to just muddle through.

By reading stories from a variety of women with varying personalities and worldviews, who experienced different sets of circumstances, you will hopefully find women or approaches or situations to which you can relate and from which you can gain ideas, insight, and inspiration. Also, as you read other women's stories, you may find out – as I did – that there are more choices available than you initially knew.

## Key themes of the book

As you've probably gathered, one of the key themes of this book is that each and every expectant mom has the opportunity to discover her unique way to be pregnant. I don't believe there is a "right" way to do pregnancy, and this book has not been written to advocate any particular choices over others.

There are many stories about choices that women made and how well those choices worked for them. That can make it feel like an endorsement, but it's not. I've tried in many cases to share the stories of women who handled situations in diametrically opposing ways. You may have strong beliefs about what choices are appropriate for pregnant women, and I would predict that the stories that reflect your point of view will validate those beliefs for you. And, you may also find yourself interested in choices you'd never considered or been exposed to before. Allow the process to be one of discovery.

The chapters include many examples of how women shifted through "shoulds" – things they felt they were supposed to do as a pregnant woman, or how they dealt with perceived pressures from others and themselves to uncover what they *actually* wanted to think and do. There is a lot of information out there about what is and is not appropriate for expectant moms. Pregnancy is a common and important process in life. People – including you – have opinions about how it should be done. You may feel very real pressure to approach aspects of pregnancy and childbirth in specific ways. One of the messages of this book, one that you'll hear repeatedly, is to identify and remove "shoulds" and pressures, and simply give yourself permission to do what, at your core, is the most aligned with your desires. I think it's about empowering an expectant mom to do what is going to make her feel most confident and comfortable. You'll see this belief expressed in many of the examples and concepts shared.

Another key message is to be super, super gentle with yourself as you're gaining clarity about and taking actions to create the pregnancy you most desire. Pregnancy is a creative and critical process, and it can be an intensely emotional time. Plus, it's brand new. You've never experienced this pregnancy before. You can't expect yourself to be perfect – or even "passable" – at something you've never done before.

Overall, it may sound like a simple approach: Learn what other pregnant women have done and choose for yourself what will work for you. Of course, it's not always that easy. Understanding what you truly want will take some processing of your thoughts and feelings to discover what truly resonates for you. Be nice to yourself along the way.

Also shared in the book is the idea that all of us have the power to choose. Now certainly, we may not get to choose all the experiences that we'll have during our pregnancy and childbirth journey. Yet, we *can* choose how we react to these experiences. We *can* choose our perspective. We *can* say how we want to "be" about our circumstances. We *can* choose what we focus on.

For example, if you're getting daily, unsolicited advice and directives from your mother-in-law, there are choices to be made. You can choose to focus on what's working, which might be that your baby will have a doting grandmother. This choice has you moving your focus away from what's not working -- that her advice is annoying you.

Another option is to look at what's not working and decide if there is something to be done about it. Perhaps you can have a conversation with your mother-in-law about her unsolicited advice. You can enlist the help of your husband to change the subject when the directives start. You can let your mother-in-law know when your choices are firm. You can choose to ignore her suggestions. The point is we get to choose our actions. We can even choose how we feel. You can actually decide whether you want to continue to be annoyed. Understanding that we are "at choice" and not complete victims of our circumstances is a key theme throughout the book.

## How to get the most from this book

As you read the ideas and stories shared in this book, look for what resonates with you and what doesn't. At times it may take a while to recognize what resonates with you. Allow for your discovery process to take whatever time is needed. Be compassionate and patient with yourself.

As you identify ideas and choices that feel like they'll work great for you, feel free to discard the rest. Just because an approach or mindset was brilliantly effective for someone else, doesn't mean it's a fit for you. You should also feel free to read a woman's account and shout out "That's complete bunk! That'll never work!" (Go ahead...she can't hear you!) Knowing what won't work for you is extremely valuable information. It gets you one step closer to knowing what you *do* want.

If there are stories that begin to make you anxious or concerned, stop reading. If there are parts of the book – or whole chapters even – that feel like they don't apply to you, don't waste your time on them. Skip around. Follow your energy and trust yourself. Truly only use what seems useful and supportive to you.

Throughout the book, there are Check Ins that invite you to pause and check in with yourself. Each Check In poses open-ended inquiries for you to answer. These are opportunities for you to step away from the stories you just read and consider what you most want to do, think, or consider in regards to an aspect of pregnancy. It's useful to take a moment – even when you think you're already really clear – to write succinctly what you're thinking and desiring. There is power in the written word and using it to declare what you want. It's also useful – even if you're not fully clear about what you want – to write your immediate thoughts and reactions. Feel free to write a "partial" response.

I'd also suggest that you be gracious with yourself when you approach a Check In. If you're not ready to answer the question, don't. If you want to come back, come back. The Check In sections are designed to remind you to consider and make note of what's resonating for you. And you might not know yet. It's all fine. Stay engaged in the inquiry. Let the questions simmer in the back of your mind for a while until you're more clear about what will work best for you. And, it's good to acknowledge that if a topic or consideration is new for you, reading a few pages about what worked for others might not be enough. You may have to "try on" some mindsets and take some actions first, and then see for yourself what fits for you. It won't be a perfect process. Use the Check In sections in the ways that best support you in the "clarifying what you want" process.

The bottom-line is to use this book however you see fit! Trust yourself. Dig in where you want to dig in. Skip what it seems you want to skip. And, look throughout for ideas and inspiration that will be specifically helpful to you. Take your unique path to discovering the pregnant you that you love.

## Acknowledgements to the women I interviewed

Of course this book would not be possible without all the women who told me their pregnancy and childbirth stories!

A very special "Thank you!" goes out to all the moms who generously gave of their time and themselves to tell me their pregnancy and childbirth experiences for this book. I am so inspired by each of you who opened up the storybooks of your life and shared authentically about what you thought and felt and experienced during pregnancy. You shared both your successes and your struggles, and I appreciate your graciousness in that.

It was an honor to be a witness to your journeys, to hear a first-hand account of what worked and inspired you and conversely concerned and dismayed you. It was so moving and motivating. You shared the "whole" story, and readers will see what it looks and feels like when a woman does it *her* way.

You're amazing. You've given the readers of this book the gift of your experience. Thank you so much.

## The use of names in this book

I interviewed over one hundred women to gather pregnancy and childbirth stories. For the most part, I've used the actual first name of the person I interviewed. At times, to make a point more succinct or powerful, I've combined several women's stories or made adjustments for clarity. When that was the case, I used a fictitious name since the story as written did not mirror one woman's real experience. There are also times when I did not receive permission to use a woman's real name, so of course, a fictitious name was used.

## Final thoughts for the readers of this book

Again, not every story included in this book is going to resonate for you – some may even baffle or scare you. I encourage you to appreciate the experience of the woman and look for yourself to determine what choices – regardless of what the other people in your life think – are going to fit best for you.

You're empowered. Make the choices that will have you loving the pregnant you.

Love and blessings to you,
Amy

# Being a Publicly
# Pregnant Person

Once you become pregnant, how you view the world shifts. You start relating to circumstances differently. You think thoughts like: "Oh, I'll be about six months pregnant at Thanksgiving." Or "I'll be nearly eight months along when my cousin gets married. What will that mean?" You might start seeing pregnant women and kids everywhere. You may begin to wonder about whether you live in a good school district. Considerations about how you'll handle weight gain, delivery, poopy diapers, or a baby who relies on you for everything come up. The thoughts and questions are unique for each person, yet the shift is universal. You are now a pregnant person, which is different than being a non-pregnant person.

Other people start to relate to you differently. Now you're a member of the Mommy Club or the Mommy to Two Kids Club or Mommy to Three or More Kids Club. Now you get the information others have been waiting to impart to you. People may start to assume that you're eager for their pregnancy and parenting stories and advice.

People – including me, including you – will have preconceived notions about how pregnant women should behave: thinking expectant moms should be quite matronly or subdued (no tabletop dancing!), or expecting them to be full of complaints and very high maintenance, or acting perpetually blissed out and happily nesting. As a pregnant woman, you are going to experience the impact of these and many other stereotypes. You may sense them from others or place certain expectations on yourself. However, always remember this: You have the opportunity to separate what society expects from pregnant women and how you feel you "should" be as a pregnant woman from how you *actually* want to be during this important time.

Whether we realize it or not, all of us absorb a lot of "shoulds" by watching those around us. You may have seen a pregnant co-worker eating healthy snacks throughout the day. Now that you're pregnant, you may think you "should" eat organic, healthy, small meals all day long. Yet, is that really going to work great for you, your schedule, your lifestyle, *and* your health? Maybe your cousin is totally enjoying the process of creating a detailed pregnancy scrapbook and is lovingly decorating the nursery with handmade treasures. You may feel you "should" do some of the same. But do you *want* to? I know that I felt I should, even though I rarely had the patience and interest in designing, shopping for, and assembling such projects. Yet instead of forcing something that I didn't enjoy, I discovered there are many different ways to document or memorialize a pregnancy. I also realized that while the idea of handmade décor for our nursery really appealed to me, I didn't have to suddenly become crafty. There were people in my family who were delighted to learn the colors of our nursery so they could make something special for our daughter!

Pregnancy is your opportunity to separate the "typical" and what you think you "should" do from what you ideally want.

It can take a bit of reflection and processing to disentangle your thought patterns, especially while pregnant, because this is a time when you are faced with decisions and circumstances you've never encountered before. You'll be thinking about yourself and others in new ways. In the midst of all this, you, uniquely, get to discover how you want to be as a pregnant person – how you want to think and feel and act. You have the opportunity to separate unwanted, external expectations from what truly resonates for *you*.

I titled this chapter "Being a *Publicly* Pregnant Person" because it is something very public that you do. Especially in later stages of pregnancy, everyone knows that you're pregnant. So that brings the added dimension for many of worrying about how others think you're doing the pregnancy thing. You may be convinced that others are on the lookout: "Is she gaining a lot of weight? Is she retaining water? Is she a cool and collected mom or is she acting like a crazy pregnant lady? Is she preparing the way we think she should?"

I would love for you (and every pregnant woman) to give yourself permission to be pregnant exactly how you would chose if you could wipe away all concerns of judgment. If you were on a deserted island with no one watching, how would you be? How would you fully express your pregnant self? You could tune into your instincts, reflect on your values, and act in ways that are in alignment with who you truly are. And, without having to assess yourself against the perceived or real expectations of others, you might be able to accept and love your pregnant self and the all choices you make.

In reality (off the deserted island), it takes self-reflection and self-awareness to unravel and quiet all the thoughts in our heads so we can hear what our hearts and our intuition are telling us. If you can do so, a profound sense of peace awaits. It's delightful to swipe away all those concerns about the "right" way to do something and confidently, purposefully step into your own unique methodology. That's available for each of you if you look for and listen to your own thoughts and feelings.

## Declaring who you want to be

So, if you could completely set aside the opinions of others (or what you *think* their opinions are), how would you ideally want to think and feel about your pregnancy? Who do you want to be as a pregnant person? For instance, do you want to be steadfastly dedicated to your health and well-being during this time and make that your primary focus? Do you want to be someone who unapologetically and powerfully asks for what she needs? Do you want to intentionally nurture creativity, authentically share your experience, or gently allow yourself to messily step into the "unknown"? Perhaps something else? Perhaps a combination of the above? The bottom line is, you can be intentional and actually choose how you want to *be* as a pregnant woman.

Check In. How do you want to "be" during your pregnancy? What phrases and adjectives do you want to use to describe your pregnant self?

It's powerful to declare this for yourself. There is a great deal of empowerment that comes with choosing your mindset and who you are "being" and not simply reacting to others and external circumstances. My wise friend Betsy says, "When you're intentional about whom you want to be, you're able to *respond* in situations instead of *react*." You're then responding with awareness and purpose, rather than reacting due to defensiveness or confusion.

Once you've declared how you want to be during your pregnancy, know that you're not going to "be" this vision of a pregnant person that you desire 100 percent of the time. You're going to mess it up. You're going to stop yourself from requesting something you know would serve you best even though you declared yourself to be someone who will always make her needs known. You're going to miss opportunities and get caught up in the day-to-day rather than making mindful choices. You're going to clam up when you're confused instead of being the unabashed, empowered pregnant woman of your dreams.

I write this not to sadden you, but to set you up for success. Know right up front that you're not going to do it perfectly. Pregnancy is something you've never done before (even if you have other children, each pregnancy is different.) You would never expect your child to start walking perfectly from step one without wobbling or falling at first. Similarly, you're going to have wobbles and falls, and they shouldn't be viewed as failures. Be gentle with yourself. Just like you're going to nurture your child when she falls and bumps her head as she's learning to walk, nurture yourself, give yourself space to acclimate to your new way of being.

## Expanding and deepening our relationships with others

When you're pregnant, there is the opportunity to intentionally shift your relationship with yourself. At the same time, whether you deliberately decide to or not, there is the possibility of expanding and deepening our relationships with others. Naturally, there is the brand new relationship you are creating with your baby, and your relationship with your partner takes on new dimensions because of pregnancy. These are paramount! Yet, we often don't immediately see or expect the evolution of other relationships in our lives.

For many of us moms-to-be, pregnancy is the beginning of a significant eye-opening process about what our mothers did. You begin to glimpse what it might have meant for her to be your mom. For you, regardless of the current relationship with your mom – whether you're close or not close; whether she's a part of your daily life or has passed on – you may now see her as a mom going through the phases of parenthood in way you never before considered or understood.

I, for example, never gave much thought about my mom having been a pregnant person until I was pregnant. Knowing that she was pregnant while my dad was building our house, I had this one visual of her pregnant, walking around the lot pointing things out to my dad. That's it. I had never thought about how she might have felt, physically or emotionally, what she was most excited about or concerned about, etc. I decided to finally ask her when I was pregnant with my daughter. She didn't always remember how it was for her back then, yet she appreciated me asking. She understood my previous lack of interest or empathy. She said, "You never fully appreciate what it's like to be a parent until you're a parent."

Of course, our moms are not the only moms out there. When you get pregnant, you enter the sisterhood of motherhood alongside all the other mothers in your neighborhood, workplace, family, groups of friends, and other communities. You now can talk with other mothers in ways you perhaps couldn't before. There are things you can express now that you are "one of them." You can gently poke fun or give a knowing glance, because you can relate. You've experienced it for yourself.

LeAnn had always thought she'd done a fairly good job of asking her parent friends about their kids, about what they thought about their young children starting sports, about loss of sleep, about things that seemed to her to be "parent" happenings and thought processes. After she gave birth to her son, she saw a whole array of thoughts and feelings she was experiencing that she never considered asking her friends about. She laughed at herself, "I really thought I was being in tune. I didn't know the half of it! I did the best I could have, certainly. My friends appreciated the conversations we had. But, we're going back now and having the *real* conversations." Her relationships with these women have developed new dimension and richness.

When you're pregnant, you are creating life. You're doing something besides paying your bills, advancing a career, or planning the neighborhood event. You're bringing a person into the world. You're nurturing a tiny, tiny being. Many people want to connect with that special power or that special period of time. They want to talk about what it's like. They want to relive their experiences of that time. The reverence for a woman with a young, precious being inside her reminds us to relate to people as people, and not as objects. It sounds harsh, yet I assert that we, as humans, can easily get into the mode of relating to each other as objects: as some "thing" that's going to cut me off on the highway, crowd into the seat next to me on the bus, take too long asking questions in front of me in line, etc. It happens. I love that a pregnancy can snap us out of it. A courageous woman nourishing another person in her belly can remind all of us, those who are pregnant and those who are observing the pregnancy of another, about the gift of life. We can realize that we are more similar than different, and that we are here to support, not compete.

Check In. What do you appreciate about the role of a pregnant woman?

## A spirit of celebration

In many cultures around the world, the pregnant mother is revered and her pregnant condition is celebrated. The kinds of celebration and ritual are as varied as the cultures in which they reside. They range from reserving the best foods for the pregnant mom and having extended family assist with housework to decorating an expectant mom's hair with flowered garlands.

Regardless of whether your culture or your family has engrained customs for honoring pregnancy or not, I invite you to consider consciously how you'd like to acknowledge the phases of the process for yourself. There are many ways to celebrate throughout a pregnancy. Do you want to capture your experience with a pregnancy journal or photo album? Marcy, for instance, had her husband take a picture of her every 4 weeks and she wrote down the key baby-related events that took place that month and the primary thoughts and feelings she was experiencing. She didn't want anything elaborate, yet she did want to *remember*. This seemed to her like a simple and meaningful way to honor and celebrate the experience.

Angie asked for specific gifts that would memorialize her pregnancy, including having excellent, high-quality pregnancy pictures taken. With these photos she could recall what she and her unborn baby looked like and honor this special time in their lives. Angie told family and close friends that she'd welcome contributions towards that experience, and her family and friends appreciated the opportunity to help her capture exactly what she wanted.

Do you want the focus of the celebration and acknowledgement to be on your baby? Maybe it feels good to have friends and family join you in the process of setting yourself up with equipment and nursery decorations and babysitting to best nurture your child.

Do you want to celebrate certain kinds of milestones? Susan, for example, decided she wanted to acknowledge the completion of each trimester. By marking the date and doing something to specifically recognize the transition, she was able to appreciate what she – and her immediate family – had accomplished and to consciously begin to declare what she'd like the next trimester to be about.

Joleen took a more comical route. She picked some milestones along the way such as "the first day in maternity pants" and "time to buy a bigger bra!" and "the day the belly button popped" as events to mark and celebrate. These, for her, were opportunities to reach out and commiserate with girlfriends and further solidify her journey into motherhood. She celebrated with her typical self-deprecating humor and found that these light-hearted milestones helped her keep these seeming "inconveniences" in perspective. She was on her way to becoming a mommy to a newborn baby and bigger pants, bigger bras, and a bigger belly button were part of that journey. She was glad that she marked these milestones with some fanfare.

The ideas shared here about how to acknowledge and celebrate pregnancy may or may not resonate for you. You have the opportunity to pick the actions that will best enable you to most enjoy and recognize the journey.

Check In. How do you want to acknowledge yourself during pregnancy and/or celebrate the process?

## Sharing the news

The role of pregnant woman, again, is one that is often played very publicly. Your changing body shape and daily habits can be clear communicators to others about the upcoming addition to your family One of your first big "public" choices is deciding when to tell other people that you're pregnant.

There are many opinions and approaches about when it's most appropriate to tell others about a pregnancy. The reasoning behind each approach varies, too. What's most important is to discover *your* rationale for how and when you want to share your news and to act in accordance to what feels right for you.

Some women share with everyone that they are pregnant right when they first learn it. There's no stopping them. The thought of following "conventional" wisdom and keeping it to themselves for the first trimester never occurs to them. The rationale usually revolves around "How could I be 'real' or connected with people when I am keeping the biggest news *ever* from them?"

That's a perfectly understandable perspective. Some would say that approach immediately creates a whole lot of people thinking about your pregnancy and intending for everything to go smoothly for you. You've got the energy of all your loved ones with you and your baby from the start!

Others don't want to share the information until after they reach week 10 or 12. And that can be fun, too. There's this wonderful secret about the miracle growing inside of them. It's like they have this mysterious little invention that they know is going to transform the world – especially their own! They may be imagining how different people will react when they share the news and considering how they will tell people. It is fun for them to have this information to themselves and have the anticipation of sharing it.

For others, perhaps because the pregnancy was unplanned or they had experienced miscarriages in the past, there may be a need to give themselves time to adjust, to process the circumstances, and to decide how they are going to proceed.

The journey is different for each of us.

Laura, given that she was a prenatal parenting educator and had spent years studying a woman's mood and imagination during pregnancy, paid close attention to her intuition during this time. Her intuition told her to keep the pregnancy private during the first few months. She didn't tell others, nor did she see a doctor. It was her joyous secret that she shared only with her husband.

Before getting pregnant, Laura didn't know that she'd feel this way. Yet afterwards, she was clear that the beginning of her pregnancy should be in stark contrast to the end of her pregnancy when everyone can't help but know you're pregnant and you're showing off a big, beautiful belly. She just followed a seemingly silly insight she was having. Laura and her husband enjoyed that private, personal time and didn't make the news public until sometime in her fourth month.

Everyone has a different rationale for sharing or not sharing the news. Many don't want to start telling others until after the likelihood of miscarriage is down to a really low probability because they think it's a jinx or they worry about the possibility of having to tell all the people in their lives that they've lost the baby. Others want to get the significant news out to loved ones because they want others to share in the "knowing" – either because they want to experience others' reactions or because they want to process their new life circumstances with others. The rationale a newly pregnant woman may have can vary.

Pay attention to yourself. Do what feels right and good for you. If it feels right to not share, don't share. If you're busting at the seams to share, shout it from the rooftops. And, you don't have to have your rationale perfectly worked out. Your rationale doesn't have to make sense to anyone else but you and your partner. You get to say what works for you.

Jen told her close friends and family about her pregnancies right away. She knew if she did have a miscarriage these were the people to whom she'd want to turn for support. So, Jen figured they might as will be along with her for the full journey. That's what made sense to her.

For me, tradition had something to do with it. My husband and I didn't tell most people until after the third month. That way, the first trimester had a different feel to it than the second trimester. In the first, we had our little, glorious secret. We were talking about what it meant to us and our immediate family. We were planning about how we'd tell others. We had the debate about finding out whether our baby was a girl or a boy. Baby names were kicked around. We talked about what kind of parents we wanted to be and how we needed to transform the house to fit another person. It was our time to be with each other and sort through our thoughts and feelings.

Another reason it worked for me to not tell everyone right away was a matter of timing. It seemed to me that my pregnancy would seem longer if we told everyone right away! Nine months sounded *so* lengthy. I wanted to break it up, spread out the pregnancy milestones, and experience three distinct trimesters. This, of course, did not actually make my pregnancy any shorter. Yet, it was part of my perspective about what worked best for me.

Your choice doesn't have to be rational. And it doesn't have to be consistent. You can do things differently in your second pregnancy if that's what you feel like. You can change your mind halfway through your first trimester. You can choose to share with some friends and not others. There doesn't have to be a rhyme or reason. Whatever works for you at this time is what is going to work for you!

Check In. When do you think you want to share the news?

Why does that timing feel good?

So, if you don't share the news with others right away, there are some other questions that can come up: "Will others somehow figure it out? Can I be authentic with people when I'm keeping this huge, pivotal piece of news from them? Am I willing to out-and-out lie? What tangle of lies am I willing to spin?"

We've all heard the stories of an insightful grandmother or friend who can "just tell" that someone is expecting. Some of us might be worried that our secret will be obvious to others based on our actions or appearance. We wonder "How will I 'fool' people into thinking I'm not pregnant when I'm not drinking alcohol at parties? Will people notice my weight gain and assume I am pregnant? What will I tell my co-workers when I'm not feeling well in the morning?"

Depending on your body type and your current habits some of these issues will be more relevant than others. And you may have others that come up for you uniquely.

## Keeping your secret secret

First, keep in mind that changes that seem huge and obvious to you might not be so monumental to those around you. When I was pregnant, I assumed everyone would notice my increased breast size. I had mistakenly thought the difference was *so* noticeable. But no, it wasn't. It was a significant change for me and my husband, but not so much for anyone else! It's a little embarrassing to admit now. Yet, sometimes it can feel like this life-altering, significant news must somehow be easily detectible by others.

If you want to keep your news secret, it helps to get clear on how you will handle it if someone asks. Debbie's approach was to be prepared with her response and to decide if she was going to admit or deny with certain groups of people. Debbie decided that she would admit it to close friends and family *if* they asked prior to her announcement. Other folks she would keep in the dark, telling them point blank that she was not pregnant if they asked her. Her rationale worked like this: She could tell them after the share date that she was sorry to have not been honest with them. She'd ask for their understanding in supporting her decision to keep her news private until she felt comfortable with widespread sharing. Debbie's experience was that people were very understanding and laughed it off, saying that they understood that many people lied about their pregnant status.

Others use a truthful yet cagey response like, "Nothing to share yet." This might seem like semantics, yet, if you are pregnant and it's before the date you plan to share with everyone, then there truly is nothing to share yet. This feels more comfortable to some than outright lying. Some take it step further with the response, "Even if I was pregnant, we wouldn't share until after the first trimester anyway."

You can find what feels genuine and appropriate for you. And, you don't have to tell everyone the same thing. If you're clear about your boundaries and don't hesitate in the moment, you have the ability to manage the conversations in the way that you wish. Many women have accomplished this.

Monica made situational decisions. If she was out with friends in a social drinking situation, she usually chose to share about her pregnancy. She made the choice to not drink any alcohol during the first half of her pregnancy, and she knew it would be too suspect for her to not have a beer or glass of wine while out. She told her friends during those social situations. She couldn't imagine lying about it and wondering all night if people believed her. This, for Monica, meant that a seemingly random group of her friends knew about her pregnancy before others, including her family. And this was okay with her. She simply informed those who were "in the know" that the news was not public yet. She asked them to keep it to themselves and explained that she was sharing because they'd probably be able to guess based on the circumstances.

Another tricky set of circumstances involves experiencing morning sickness around people with whom you don't yet want to share your pregnant status. Jennifer felt really concerned about this one. Mid-morning, like clockwork she'd need to go to the bathroom and throw up. She felt like it was so obvious to everyone at her workplace. She started varying her morning schedule so she didn't meet with the same people every day at 10:00 a.m. Outside of that, she wasn't sure what to do. She just worried that others were catching on and were simply too polite to say anything to her. She found out afterwards that no one was the wiser, so changing up her schedule and not bringing attention to her bathroom visits by making up false excuses had worked to keep her secret secret.

Other women have felt concerned about some co-workers coming to their own conclusions and have used an approach similar to Monica's. Instead of having their news be rumored at the water cooler, they decided to share in confidence about their pregnancies with close co-workers. Most people feel honored to be part of the chosen few who know the significant news before the rest of the world and will probably help you keep your secret.

Find the approach that will work and feel good for you.

Check In. If you choose to keep your pregnancy secret for a time, how will you do that?

How will you respond if someone asks you if you are pregnant?

## Your emotions and others' reactions

Eventually, the time will come when you will be telling people that you are pregnant.

When you're sharing news that is this important, it's natural that you want people to respond in a way that feels supportive to you and matches your emotional state. If you're excited, you want others to be excited. If you're cautiously optimistic, you may want others to be cautiously optimistic, too. If you're nervous, you want people to be supportive.

And the reality is that you are probably experiencing a range of emotions that change at unexpected times. This is often one of the most surprising elements of the first trimester. I've talked with many women who expected to feel simply excited and overjoyed upon finding out that they were pregnant. And, instead, they found themselves also experiencing fear, anxiety, uncertainty, pride, love, and other emotions along with that excitement and joy. The emotional reaction to learning you're growing a baby inside of you is complex. You may not know how you want others to respond when how you feel shifts from day to day or hour to hour.

Spend some time with your own thoughts and feelings. Know where you're at in the emotional range. When you're clear about how you feel, you tend to radiate your needs more clearly, even if they change frequently. Knowing and accepting your feelings will enable you to more readily recognize what you need in terms of emotional support.

Others may or may not intuitively know how you'd best like them to respond. Understand that this may be the case, and feel free to tell or guide others as to what you need from them. If someone starts expressing concerns that you don't want to hear, you can simply let them know, "I just want your support and enthusiasm at this time." Or you can be more proactively prescriptive, letting others know specifically what you'd most like to hear from them.

Check In. What emotions are you experiencing?

What kind of response do you most want from others?

As you're telling others your news and perhaps asking for some support, you will also encounter the opinions, outlooks, and emotions of others that will show up in how they react to you. These might be related to you and your news, or they might be related to the person's own experiences or views of pregnancy and pregnant women in general.

For instance, I used to think that pregnant women were wimpy, preoccupied with themselves, and apt to have physical and emotional issues all the time. Mind you, the pregnant women that I had interacted with up until that time weren't that way. My friends had been amazingly able – I see in hindsight – to focus on many other subjects and not have our interactions during their pregnancies be solely focused on them and their growing bellies. They were not wimpy or riddled with issues. Yet, still, that kind of general stereotype lingered and I was applying the stereotype subconsciously to pregnant women I saw in the course of the day who I didn't know. Now, I can see that this view had much more to do with my insecurities about being able to handle pregnancy gracefully than it did with the actual behaviors of the women around me. I was afraid that I'd be wimpy and needy and complainy, so that was what I was projecting on others.

The reactions you receive from others may have much more to do with their general outlook, than anything to do with your specific situation.

## ✽ OKAY, LET'S BE REAL… ✽ ✽ ✽ ✽ ✽ ✽ ✽ ✽ ✽

### People are making assumptions about MY pregnancy!

It's easy for people to assume that if someone is married and over the age of 22 that pregnancy is good news. It can also be easy to assume that if someone is unmarried, a teenager, just lost her job, or had a baby 3 months ago, pregnancy is bad news. Although it's easy to make these assumptions, they aren't always true, and it does not feel good to be on the receiving end of an erroneous assumption!

People should check their assumptions! They ought to ask a question or two before they start providing sympathy you don't want or before they start overwhelming you with enthusiasm you don't share.

When this happens, we can be left feeling like we're the ones who have to clarify *their* misunderstanding. Otherwise, we're in essence confirming their inaccurate perspective. It's a frustrating situation in which you might feel like you have to explain and defend.

Instead, it would be nice if others would verify their assumptions before verbalizing them. Or, ultimately, not even make the assumption to begin with!

Yet, we know, people are not perfect. So, when faced with an erroneous assumption, we might need to scrounge up as much graciousness as we possibly can , grit our teeth, and

✿ try to remember that we've all probably made an inaccurate ✿
✿ assumption at some point.                                    ✿

✿ ✿ ✿ ✿ ✿ ✿ ✿ ✿ ✿ ✿ ✿ ✿ ✿ ✿ ✿ ✿ ✿ ✿ ✿ ✿ ✿

## Reacting to the spotlight

Some women love the attention-getting aspects pregnancy can bring. Others don't. Some only enjoy certain types of attention or the spotlight in certain circumstances. A pregnant belly can attract streams of curious questions, and there are also special events that occur just because someone is pregnant.

Baby showers are one of the phenomena that can create wanted or unwanted attention. You might be part of a family where traditional "guess the circumference of the pregnant belly, play baby word search, and eat cake" baby shower is the expected course of action, no questions asked. That might be alright with you, or you may cringe at even the idea of being center stage at such an event. You can look at whether you're willing to go along with what's expected and desired by others or if you're willing to upset some important people in your life in order to do what you want. Or, if you can, come to some sort of compromise. It is your pregnancy and you can choose how it's acknowledged and celebrated. And that is not necessarily an argument for disregarding the expectations and desires of others. It may be really appealing to you to have your loved ones be happy and harmonious during your pregnancy, and having a traditional shower may be part of the formula that achieves that.

It's up to you to process your thoughts and desires around the idea of a baby shower and choose what's best for you. That is what Jennifer did.

"When Aunt Betty starts planning and sharing her ideas around a potential baby shower, ask for a moment to think about what'll work," she advised. You could ask for time to check on some dates and use that reprieve to consider what you're willing to engage in.

For Jennifer, this pause gave her the time to accept for herself what was going to happen before the shower took on a life of its own. She was able to make a conscious decision and then be responsible for it. She could tell herself, "I chose this," rather than being a victim the whole time or rolling her eyes. Now, Jennifer did have some specific requests, including a "no games" rule and that the format of the shower be a casual potluck. With those parameters, she let her family members planning the event run with the rest.

For Gretchen the choice looked different. The aunts in her husband's large family offered to throw a baby shower. Even though Gretchen didn't enjoy being the center of attention in these kinds of circumstances, she also didn't feel she could say a flat out "No" to their generous offer. Instead, she focused on their great intentions and desires to celebrate the arrival of her new baby. Gretchen didn't make any specific requests and on the day of the event, Gretchen included her sister-in-law, who was a few months less pregnant than she was, in the majority of pictures. It was Gretchen's way of being more comfortable in the spotlight. She chose to share it.

Erin wasn't concerned about the BBQ-style shower her family would host. She was, instead, surprised to find herself the focus of every family gathering during her pregnancy. Her aunts, uncles, and cousins would assemble and pepper her with questions: "How are you feeling? Is it a boy or a girl? Where are you delivering? Why did you choose that hospital? Isn't there one closer?"

Depending on her temperament (and the line of questioning), Erin sometimes enjoyed and sometimes resented the attention. It made her feel a little like Dr. Jekyll and Mr. Hyde.

Erin realized in hindsight that she had handled the interactions perfectly. She glowed in the spotlight and animatedly answered questions when she wanted. And, at other times, she deflected the inquiries changing the topic to others' lives and even walked away when she wasn't in the mood to be the focus of the conversation. She did what she wanted in the moment and was glad she hadn't forced herself to have a perfectly consistent type of response.

Check In. How do you want to leverage and/or deflect the spotlights that might shine on you during pregnancy?

## Unplanned pregnancy

So what happens when you find yourself pregnant when you weren't trying? How do you handle that publicly and privately?

Shannon had an unplanned pregnancy. She was 17 and a senior in high school when she got pregnant. When she first found out, she didn't know how she was going to handle it privately, let alone publicly. For the first several months, Shannon hid out. She was petrified and was discovering that her boyfriend was not going to be a partner in the process. It took her some time to get her bearings.

After experiencing a great deal of fear and overwhelm, she discovered her intestinal fortitude. She tapped into levels of personal strength that she didn't even know she had and discovered what her commitments were. She was committed to completing her education. She was committed to debunking the stereotype prevalent in her hometown about pregnant teenagers dropping out of school and giving up on their life dreams. She was committed to taking good care of her baby.

It took courage to generate these convictions, to carve a new and different path for herself, and to do it all publicly. Her town and other students would be watching. Shannon said it really came to the forefront the first day she had to wear maternity clothes to school and face her classmates who all knew she had been "dumped" by her boyfriend. There was a suit of armor she wore that day that she believes was her maternal instinct.

The girl who had the locker next to Shannon would ask every day, especially as Shannon grew bigger, "When are you quitting school?

When are you leaving?" Shannon would reply, "I don't know what you're talking about." Quitting school did not line up with Shannon's commitments.

Looking back, Shannon could see that she spent a significant amount of time in overwhelm and fear. But spending the time there, allowed her to get to a place where she could be clear about her commitments and how she wanted to be during her pregnancy and as a mother. In telling her story, she didn't apologize for the time spent in anxiety and worry and shame. She doesn't think she should have done it differently or berate herself for not being able to do it differently. She just made sure that she came out of that time with her convictions clear.

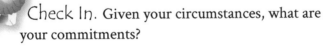

Check In. Given your circumstances, what are your commitments?

## Viewing pregnancy as an opportunity, not a burden

I can tell you that there was a time when I couldn't imagine considering the prospect of being pregnant as an "opportunity" of any kind. I initially regarded pregnancy as a burden. Pregnancy was a time when people would be watching how much weight I gained, how I dealt with shifting hormones, and what kinds of decisions I made regarding my care and delivery. I wasn't sure I could "do" pregnancy well, and I feared I was going to fail with an audience.

Then, despite my cynicism and fears, when we first were considering when and if to become pregnant, I found myself initiating the conversations with my husband and having more well-thought out perspectives than he. I kept wondering, "When is my husband going to get as engaged as I am?" I'm used to having a 50/50 shared partnership. When is he going to contribute at a 50% level in this area?

Well it took me a little while, but I eventually got it that "I'm the mother." It's going to be my body that houses our baby, my breasts from which the baby might eat, my motherly "make our house a home" instinct that's going to bring us together as a family. I have to be the mom. There are ways that I will be engaged that dad can't be.

I adjusted to this perspective and spent some time processing it. When I needed pregnancy to be a 50/50 project with my husband, I was still relating to it as a burden. When I shifted my thinking to "I have to be the mom" I could see that I had specific roles that my husband couldn't take on even if he wanted. Then, I made the next shift in my journey. I realized I wouldn't want to give up this responsibility, this privilege. That's when my perspective shifted to "I *get* to be the mom." I get to be the one who's pregnant, who nurtures our baby, and who literally nourishes him or her with my own body.

For Julie, the ability and the opportunity to be pregnant – to be the one who carried the baby, housed the baby, got to feel the baby kick and move around inside her, and got to be the one who literally nurtured the baby before he was born and for over a year afterward (because Julie chose to breastfeed for that time) – was a privilege. Her baby thrived and developed solely on what she as his mother provided. It was quite an awesome prospect and experience for her. She felt good about her babies (she has two) being healthy and well-developed under her care. She did that. No one else did. She created and sustained life. It's a miraculous, amazing occurrence that we're often not present to.

It's hard for me now to go back to the thoughts and feelings I had when I was confused about how the role of motherhood would fit into my 50/50 marriage partnership. To relate to pregnancy like a burden rather than a privilege seems so foreign now. Yet, it was quite real and magnified by the idea that I'd be struggling in "public."

If you're in a place of viewing pregnancy as an inconvenience or obligation, give yourself the space to experience and process that. You may not ever move beyond it. I've interviewed a number of women who did not overall enjoy being pregnant. Trying to say publicly that you enjoy an experience, when you clearly do not, will bring about additional struggle. Instead, you can do your best to let it be. You can focus on the choices that work best for you and deal with circumstances in the most empowering way you can. That's all any of us are doing anyway!

Check In. What do you currently view as a pregnancy-related inconvenience or burden?

What opportunities do you see for your pregnancy?

## OKAY, LET'S BE REAL…

Sometimes people say <u>too</u> much!

Okay, let's be real! Sometimes – and maybe you've experienced this – people can feel an amazing freedom to say whatever they like to pregnant women! They provide unsolicited advice and say whatever occurs to them with no "filtering." And often, this is not at all helpful!

Here are examples of the *so* not helpful things people will say:

- Total stranger at a coffee shop: "No, you can't use sugar substitute. Don't do that!"

- To an expectant mother of twins: "Wow, you're so small. Are you sure the babies are okay?"

- To a woman keeping down only one meal a day due to nausea: "You should eat more."

- "Wow, are you getting big!" (This is said frequently!)

- From a stranger at a business networking event: "I'm an intuitive and I'm picking up a bad vibe. When is your next doctor's appointment? It's not life threatening, but something is going on with the baby."

- "I've heard awful things about your doctor."

- "That's the last place I'd choose to deliver a baby."

What is it about a pregnant belly that gives people free license to let their opinions be known? Who knows?

✻   What there is to know is this: Whatever crazy thing they   ✻
✻   say... their words say more about them than you. Their   ✻
✻   comments reflect *their* thoughts and potential insecurities.   ✻
✻   They need not be yours.   ✻

✻ ✻ ✻ ✻ ✻ ✻ ✻ ✻ ✻ ✻ ✻ ✻ ✻ ✻ ✻ ✻ ✻ ✻

## Patterned conversations

When we are expecting, we are going to encounter many "typical" or patterned conversations with people as a publicly pregnant person. It might come from friends, family, or complete strangers.

Every pregnant woman gets asked the same handful of questions, seemingly every day. They can be basic: "When are you due?" "Is this your first?" "Are you having a boy or a girl?" Some get more specific and personal: "Where are you delivering?" "Are you going to use drugs or give birth naturally?" Pregnancy is a very public endeavor (at least in the last trimester) and some people think it's rude to *not* say something about it. So, know you're going to get the questions. And, know you can answer them however you want.

Personally, I enjoyed people asking me questions. I loved sharing that I was having a girl (and in my second pregnancy, a boy) and what name we picked out. Then I could introduce them to McKenzie, or tell them how I enjoyed her having an identity already. Often, I would acknowledge, "I know many people make different choices about finding out the gender and picking and sharing baby names." This invited folks to share about choices they had made or experienced with their family and friends. For me, it was a great conversation starter. This became even more apparent at the first networking event that I went to after McKenzie was born. I quickly realized that I didn't have my pregnant belly conversation starter anymore! I was going to have to initiate conversation with my mouth. My pregnant shape wouldn't do it for me any longer. It was only then that I fully realized how much I appreciated having the freedom and implicit invitation to talk about something so precious and important in my life.

Not everyone appreciates the direct questions, of course. This can be particularly true when others ask about choices that are yours alone to make like finding out the gender of the baby or where you're going to deliver. You may not want to hear all the advantages to finding out gender ahead of time, if that's not your choice. You may not want to explain why you feel comfortable giving birth at home to someone you just met. Even the most innocuous questions like "When are you due?" can open you up to receiving people's opinions when they comment that you're "so small" or "so big" relative to your due date.

Know that there are ways to deal with these situations and share only what you'd like to without having to scream, "It's none of your damn business!"

When people would comment on Marsha's pregnancy or ask a question like "How are you feeling?" she would respond (talking quickly and jokingly) with something like, "This is my first, I'm due in May, and we'll find out gender at the birth, much to the dismay of our family. I've answered these questions so many times, I've got the streamlined response! What is new in your life?" And, she'd turn the conversation back to the other person. For the most part, Marsha was able to share only what she wanted to share and then steer the focus onto the other person. Now, sometimes the person couldn't shift topics that quickly. For example, they'd follow up on the "to the dismay of our family" comment. Still, she had fun playing with it and seeing what felt authentic, social, and polite, yet within her comfort level of what she wanted to share.

It can also be easy to feel pressure to always be upbeat and happy, to say that everything's going great and that you are completely excited about what's happening and what you've chosen. But the reality is that sometimes it's not going great or you have doubts or you aren't entirely secure in your choices. That's a normal part of the process.

I've coached women to answer people honestly when asked about how they're feeling – even if they're not, in that moment, focusing on something positive. That's not to say you should share anything that you don't feel okay sharing. Yet, this can be a place for stretching ourselves and seeing what it would feel like to give a fully truthful response. "I feel irritable and cranky and like I have no control over it." "I'm not sure how I feel about having a boy! They are rambunctious and smelly and unfamiliar to me." The person you are talking to might freeze up and not know how to respond. They might not be used to blunt truths shared like this. Or, they might be totally ready to hear what you're saying and you'll find empathy and useful thoughts where you didn't expect them. You never know what you'll get in return unless you put your true feelings out there.

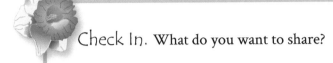

Check In. What do you want to share?

What do you not want to share?

## Having the "whole" conversation

In Debra's family, they had always talked openly about pregnancy and birth, and were particularly proud about not shying away from discussing the messy process of birth. Delivery stories were passed down from generation to generation. Since Debra was a little girl, she'd known that her great-grandmother gave birth to eight kids at home. Debra's great-grandmother would work on the farm all day and when she felt that it was about time, she'd go into her kitchen, dangle herself over the kitchen sink and give birth there. The older siblings knew what was going on and, in some instances, helped catch their new younger brother or sister as they were born. Birth was not something to hide from the family. It was not considered too messy or intimate to be shared.

Debra felt this openness had benefited her family in many ways. She believed her female relatives had less trepidation about their pregnancies because they'd been exposed to what happens and were not overwhelmed by "unknowns." She saw male relatives actively support their pregnant wives. Familiarity and exposure created comfort and confidence in her family.

In Jenny's case, she wished she'd been more informed about what was *really* going to happen, including the unexpected, confusing, dirty, awkward, and gross parts.

After Jenny delivered her son at home in a blowup swimming pool, she was helped to an air mattress where she then delivered the placenta. In hindsight, she said she wasn't at all prepared for the process of delivering the placenta. For her, it was painful, strange, and confusing.

Jenny had always been aware that there were aspects of pregnancy and birth that "we" as a society don't talk about and this experience of delivering her placenta just underlined that for her. So, in an effort to capture the totality of her birth experience, Jenny took pictures of the pool after the birth of her son. She captured the multi-colored water. She admitted it was weird and she wasn't sure what she'd do with the pictures. Yet, something profound and extremely important had taken place there. She wanted to memorialize that. It was a beautiful, miraculous event *and*...it was human and messy and involved bodily excretions.

Now, this might not at all be something you're comfortable looking at or discussing. That's totally fine and that's really good for you to know. You want to do what works for you. And, I see an opportunity to expand what gets shared in mainstream conversations to help dissipate the feelings of confusion and shame that you can feel when you're grappling with something completely foreign or new. When you've never heard anyone talk about what you're experiencing, you can assume that what's occurring is obviously embarrassing or shameful or weirdly rare. Right? That's why no one talks about it!

When we're feeling gross and confused, for example, about this unidentifiable discharge on our underwear "Is it the mucus plug already? Is it normal to just have some ongoing discharge during the third trimester? Am I peeing my pants a little bit all the time?" It can be the *last* thing we want to talk about with people. My desire for women to share stems from not wanting anyone to feel gross or ashamed of something that's simply normal and natural.

You'll encounter weird or disconcerting aspects of pregnancy and birth. That's a given. You can choose to hide these aspects from others, feeling confused, ashamed, and alone. Or you can courageously share about them and discover that it's not weird or concerning, or that you are at least not alone in those feelings.

Check In. What is difficult to accept? What feels unnatural, weird, annoying, or gross?

What is surprisingly easy to accept?

Today, more and more pregnant moms are being very intentional about what they are creating and are sharing their full stories, including the good, the disappointing, and the miraculous! For some, the messy, bodily excretion-type aspects of the pregnancy experience might be the most disconcerting and difficult to talk about. Others take this in stride, yet might find different aspects to be uncomfortable, silly, or embarrassing. There can be great value in talking freely and openly.

## Share your experience

One of the key themes of this book – as you're probably well aware by now – is to discover the approaches and methods that work best for you during your pregnancy and give yourself permission to do things your way. As you see, I'm breaking pattern with that in this chapter and suggesting a specific action: share with others about what you're experiencing during your pregnancy.

I specifically suggest talking to others because it creates an access point to enabling others to support us. Too often we feel that we're alone, that no one has experienced what we're experiencing. We think that we're flawed in some unique way and that we're the only ones who aren't able to effectively deal with whatever issue is bothering us. We haven't heard anyone else we know talk about their concerns of becoming a mom or getting hemorrhoids or obsessively enjoying their bigger boobies or any other seemingly significant or superficial thing that we're chewing on. We're too embarrassed or too proud or too "something" to bring it up. It takes courage to share openly. It's an effort that requires a willingness to be vulnerable and open ourselves up to scorn, gossip, or judgment.

In talking with hundreds of women about pregnancy, I have heard time and again of the relief and practical ideas that we can get when we finally admit the one thing that we've been keeping under wraps and not letting the public see. The people we open up to might not always have shared that same specific thought. Yet, they've had their own flavor of it or they might simply appreciate being the confidante that you trusted.

It is such a gift to generate this kind of dialogue. You have the opportunity for cathartic relief, for getting some perspective around something that is consuming you, for getting concrete ideas that you can take action on, and for providing a space where the other person can get the same. They get to know that they're not alone, either! It's truly amazing. I've experienced it and I've gotten the opportunity to witness it through the telling of other people's stories.

Does it ever backfire? Sure, it can. You might want to set the other person up for the type of conversation you want to have. You may say something like, "There's something I want to share with you, and I feel nervous and vulnerable about it. I'm not ready to laugh about it or trivialize it. Can I share?"

I know, for me, there were a few thoughts and concerns that I had spent a good deal of time being obsessed and repressed about. I was terrified that I would be seen as a freak or superficial or self-centered. And, every time I pushed myself into opening up, I was met with compassion, concern, or suggestions. It wasn't always the "perfect" response. I had to prepare myself for that. I had some people laugh more than I wanted when I shared about my concern about getting hemorrhoids. I had another person tell me, "It's inevitable. There's nothing you can do." I didn't enjoy that comment in the moment, yet it ultimately had me seeking out a number of women who pushed during delivery for a long time and never got hemorrhoids. I was able to believe that I, too, didn't *have* to get hemorrhoids.

I want us all to have the experience of knowing that we are not alone. This is available most powerfully by sharing your thoughts and feelings. True to the book's theme, how you choose to share can look myriad ways. You could talk to a coach inside a confidential relationship, you could talk to everyone and anyone who will listen, you could open up to a small select group of trusted friends, etc. The "how" is not as important as the act of doing it.

Trust yourself. Seek out people you trust the most, the ones you think will be able to engage in the conversation in the way you want them to. It doesn't have to be your best friend or your mom or your partner. It could be them or it could be a co-worker or coach with whom you have a connection. The advice is to check any hesitation you have in this arena and stretch yourself to share more than you might normally and naturally. The results might not be perfect, yet they can be extremely useful.

Check In. What do you know in your heart of hearts would be cathartic, relieving, useful to share with someone?

With whom will you share?

## ✸ Being a Publicly Pregnant Person

Being the publicly pregnant person you want to be starts with knowing your commitments. It takes continually examining your thoughts and feelings to discover the choices you want to make and how you want to handle certain circumstances. Sometimes this only takes a moment of reflection. Other times this takes longer. Other times situations will crop up on you and you won't know how you want to handle them.

You won't do it perfectly. It's great to learn from mistakes. And, you can always change your mind.

* It's powerful to declare for yourself how you want to "be" as a pregnant person.

* You get to choose when and how you share about your pregnancy. You can decide what you want to share with others throughout your pregnancy.

* Your perspectives affect how others interact with you.

* Even if you didn't choose a particular set of circumstances, you can choose your commitments inside of them.

* There are incredible joys and opportunities available in the experience of being pregnant.

* You're not alone. The more you're able to share, the more you'll realize you're not alone.

Check In. What, for you, are the keys to enjoying being a publicly pregnant person?

# Embracing Your Feelings

Being pregnant! How do you feel about it? Depending on your journey to this place, you may feel excited, relieved, overjoyed, blessed, disappointed, shocked, scared, overwhelmed, nervous, inadequate, empowered, peaceful, or myriad other emotions. It's likely you are experiencing a nice confusing mix of the aforementioned. It's also natural to have heightened emotions during a pregnancy. These new and varying emotions can provide access to important insights about yourself.

To illustrate the intensity and range of feelings that might come up, let's look at the possible layers to the seemingly simple question: How do you feel about being pregnant?

A natural first reaction, when you're asked about how it feels to be pregnant, is to explain what it feels like to know you're going to have a baby, to know you're going to be a mom to an infant. We tend to answer more about how we're feeling about being a *parent*, rather than how we're reacting to the idea that we're *pregnant*. And, of course, there are probably a lot of things you are feeling and could say about being a parent! Yet, how does it feel to know you're *pregnant*, that you are now a pregnant person and will be for many coming months? The response may be the same: excited, relieved, overjoyed, blessed, disappointed, shocked, etc. Yet, the question is different, isn't it?

There are other potential nuances to the question as well. What does it feel like *right now* to be pregnant? How do you feel knowing you'll be pregnant for the next nine or so months? How do you feel about the changes you'll go through physically, mentally, and emotionally during your pregnancy? How do you feel about childbirth?

The many possible considerations of this simple question: "How do you feel about being pregnant?" demonstrate the intensity and range of emotions we might experience throughout the pregnancy journey. There are strong reactions and different feelings you might articulate for each of the different nuances to the question. These are the layers of inquiry that you'll be considering or living with while pregnant.

## Emotions are a gift

Pregnancy gives you a lot to process. You're going to find yourself experiencing a whole range of emotions and physical sensations that are new and ever-changing throughout your pregnancy. More than anything else, it's important to understand that having a variety of emotions, or experiencing emotions that you didn't expect to feel, is normal and natural. These are not something to hide from or try to pretend aren't there.

You're engaging with sets of questions and deliberations as a pregnant woman that you've never contemplated before and maybe never even *thought* of contemplating before. Naturally, all these new questions and things to think about are going to have new feelings associated with them. And you may find that feelings shift and change, their intensity ebbing and flowing at different points in your pregnancy. Many women experience this. You are not alone.

It's okay to feel overwhelmed and over-taken by emotions at times. Who wouldn't? Know that you can deal with them, that you can unravel them bit-by-bit. You can deal with them one at a time.

And, if you're thinking that you haven't felt emotional and don't expect to, remember that unaffected, peaceful, apathetic, grounded, and withdrawn are also ways you can feel. You can learn from both your seemingly "positive" and "negative" emotions. Throughout this chapter, we'll look at ways to allow your feelings to be what they are, without trying to change or wish away any uncomfortable emotions, and to allow them to be a guide for you.

Check In. How do you feel? What are your most prevalent feelings right now?

The emotions that come up during pregnancy are an important means of personal growth. We can always learn from our feelings and this is especially the case during pregnancy. As we begin to parent the baby in our womb, there are new ways of being that we have to adapt to, there are new ways of looking at the world that we are trying on. Our feelings let us know what actions are aligned with our values and how we want to be as a parent, and they let us know when things are not jelling for us. Emotions during this time are a gift. They show us where to look and what we want to understand to be the most powerful and empowered human being and mother we can be.

Certain kinds of "hooks" we encounter during pregnancy are designed so we can deal with issues prior to being responsible for a baby outside the womb. A "hook" is a concern or anxiety that takes over our thoughts and feelings for a bit. When you're hooked, you can feel caught in a swirl without knowing how to move forward literally and figuratively. Everyone has hooks and they look different for everyone. A hook may be a physical characteristic that feels unnatural or uncomfortable, it may be medical practitioners talking about your weight gain, or people assuming any emotion you demonstrate is heightened due to hormones, or worrying that you're getting more forgetful, or any number of other circumstances that make you feel exposed and uncomfortable in a way that you can't shake.

When you pay attention to what your hooks are, and when you find ways to work through them, you're not just solving your problem in the moment, you are teaching yourself how you're going to deal with similar situations in the future.

It's a nice design in many ways. You're pregnant for nine months. During this time, you're a parent to a baby that is seemingly protected in your belly, and because you're already a parent, your parental lessons-to-learn can get kicked up before you're involved with the logistics of caring for a newborn.

Natalie, for example, was infuriated - and clearly hooked - when her female co-worker would insinuate that Natalie was over-reacting to a situation due to hormones. She would want to argue and deny that hormones had anything to do with her conviction. This, in her co-worker's eyes, just validated the idea that Natalie was overly emotional. Natalie finally gave up trying to change her co-worker's perspective. She realized that there were going to be times as a parent that she was going to get worked up on behalf of her child and her family. And, she wanted that to be okay. She didn't want to have to convince others that her reaction was appropriate or justified. There were going to be times when people would think she was over-reacting or maybe not responding strongly enough. She decided in her pregnancy that she was not going to spend her time, as a parent, justifying her emotions to others. Pregnancy can be the perfect time for you to discover how you want to approach certain circumstances, how you want to think and act as a parent.

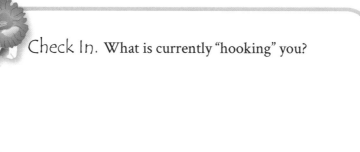

Check In. What is currently "hooking" you?

Some of the emotions we experience are really fun and fulfilling like excitement, feeling special, and pride. Others may be disconcerting, strange, and anxiety provoking. Whatever they are, it's important that you let them in and not be tempted to brush aside the highest of the highs or the most unsettling of the lows. It can be easy to not trust the euphoria and want to resist the uncomfortable or confusing. There is something to be learned from it all. There is a way in which our capacities are expanded on both ends of the spectrum. Being able to be with our emotions and process them effectively is a skill and practice that will serve us the rest of our lives. As parents, there will continue to be highs and lows that we'll experience on this journey with our children.

## Heightened emotions

There are many factors that can create intense highs and lows during our pregnancies. There are significant changes occurring emotionally, mentally, and physically. We are carrying around a very precious being in our bellies. People are watching us and noting how we're dealing with changes in our lives. These are circumstances ripe with the possibility of feeling new and different and intense emotions.

Becky, as a mother of three kids, noticed heightened anxiety and desperate feelings that she wasn't able to fully protect her unborn baby. She noticed them each time she was pregnant, and had spent a lot of time thinking that she didn't want to feel that way. She wanted to be a calm and assuring mother.

In her third pregnancy, it finally dawned on her: This need to protect and the anxiety around failing to fully protect were *never* going away. She realized that whether her kids were in her belly, were toddlers, or were teenagers, Becky was not going to be able to protect them against every possible concern or danger. For her, it was a relief to actually accept that these feelings were there and they were going to be a part of motherhood. It wasn't "wrong" or "inappropriate" for her to feel this way. She loved her kids, wanted them to always be safe, so she was going to feel vulnerable and anxious at times.

By trying to get rid of the emotions, they took more of a hold on her. When she was able to acknowledge them and let them be, she felt some relief. Becky eventually felt glad that she experienced these heightened emotions during pregnancy. It allowed her to increase her ability to be with the seemingly out-of-control feelings to protect. She knew this would serve her well as her children grew.

Elizabeth was amazed how things "got to her" more during her pregnancy. She viewed all world events through a different and more passionate lens because this was the world into which she was now bringing a baby. She'd hear news reports involving violence and she'd react in her gut. She didn't want humans harming other humans. It disappointed her in a profound way.

Also, the summer Olympics took place during Elizabeth's pregnancy and she'd find herself moved to tears event after event. It was an emotional delight for her to see countries come together for international competitive sport. She was touched by the way athletes dedicated years of training to a sport they loved in order to compete and make their countries proud. She'd never before reacted to the news or to the Olympics in this way, and it initially made her feel weak and overly dramatic.

For a time, Elizabeth tried to avoid anything that might cause intense emotion for her. Then, she realized that avoidance was not an approach she wanted for her life! She shifted her thinking and started to commend herself for being completely engaged in circumstances and experiencing her emotions fully. She was a mommy now and she was feeling differently at times. This was okay. She could choose to own and respect her feelings.

Check In. In what ways are your emotions heightened?

How can you view these heightened emotions in a positive light?

## OKAY, LET'S BE REAL…

I don't want to be told how to feel!

When you're pregnant, you're dealing with a whole new view of your world and are, at times, struggling to keep up with your ever-changing thoughts and emotions. What you don't need is for others to tell you how you should feel!

Pregnant women have been told:

- "Don't worry about it. Women have been doing this forever."

- "You should just feel blessed."

- "Remember how happy you'll be when you're holding your newborn baby."

- "You're over-reacting. Everything will be fine."

There are times when one of these statements is the last thing you want or need to hear.

You may even know that what the other person is saying is true, yet, in that moment, you're feeling what you're feeling and there's no reason to feel differently.

I think you should give yourself at least two free passes during your pregnancy to shout out "Don't tell me how to feel!" and then try to not feel bad about the shouting… ☺

## Anxieties about your changing body being on display

During pregnancy, our bodies change for all to see. Our boobs, bellies, and other areas are getting bigger. We've all heard friends gossiping about how so-and-so's hips widened. Or about how much weight that one gained.

It's all true, hips widen and weight goes up and there's nothing wrong with it. It's pretty much part of the process. Yet, there are people talking about hips and weight and other ways pregnant woman look different over time! Our physical changes are out there for everyone to see.

In her first pregnancy, Melinda experienced a physical characteristic that felt so vulnerable to her: her belly button pop out. It was just so out there and apparent when it popped. Melinda said it was like an obvious nipple or a sign that she had gotten "that" big. It bothered her. During her second pregnancy, her belly button popped out months earlier than with her first child.

She decided she had to give up feeling embarrassed. She didn't want to spend months trying to figure out which clothes would hide the protrusion. And it was summertime and she was hot, so she didn't want to consider adding more layers. Melinda got defiant about it. She thought, "Here it is. My belly button popped out super early. Take a look!" She became proud of it. It was amazing what was possible when she stopped resisting the vulnerability and embraced it.

Now, I know dealing with a belly button pop out may not sound like a significant example of heightened emotions. It may seem so superficial and not important in the big scheme of things. And, Melinda had those thoughts, too. She made it worse by trying to tell herself that she shouldn't feel embarrassed and worked up about something like that. But she was.

Vanessa was always known as someone who was full of energy. She kept herself in good shape, and she was constantly on the move. She enjoyed the intensity of her busy work and personal life. So when she moved into her third trimester and found herself completely winded after hustling up a flight of stairs, she hated how it felt. She felt so pathetic and feeble and not like herself. She took pride in being known as having unlimited energy and here she was clearly facing "limits." It was humbling. Vanessa tried to keep bounding up the stairs at work, tried to keep up her previous pace, and got more and more frustrated and down on herself. It was impacting her usual positive outlook in life. She begrudgingly admitted that she needed to make changes.

The next day at work, she took the elevator. A co-worker made the comment, "Vanessa is taking the elevator?! I can't believe it. I thought you were made of energy." Vanessa forced herself to laugh and replied that she was indeed made of energy, just more of it was going to internal baby making that others couldn't see. It became her go-to phrase when someone commented that Vanessa wasn't displaying her trademark energy in ways they were used to. Vanessa found ways to laugh off others' reactions and acknowledge herself for the amount of energy it took to grow a person and make lungs and eyelids and other body parts. And, after some time, she even stopped being embarrassed by how winded she was after climbing a flight of stairs.

Check In. How are you feeling about the changes to your body?

What, if anything, feels embarrassing or vulnerable to you?

## Being at the mercy of your body

In her second pregnancy, Leslie was screened for diabetes and was diagnosed, for a second time, at about 14 weeks. She was, once again, on a restrictive diet and this time the diagnosis came earlier in her pregnancy. Since Leslie was a fighter and someone who didn't like to take "No" for an answer, she found it challenging to tell herself that she couldn't have a cookie or a Frappucino or any of the items now banished from her diet. She felt trapped.

This feeling of being at the mercy of her body began when she first got her gestational diabetes diagnosis in the diabetic educator's office. She cried hard and was telling the educators how difficult it would be for her to work this into her life. Later, she recalled what a cancer patient once said, which was, "I have cancer, but cancer doesn't have me."

In that moment in the office, it felt to Leslie as if diabetes completely had her. It felt dismal and overwhelming and horribly restrictive. It took Leslie about a week and a half of feeling disappointed and frustrated and angry until she was able to shake off those emotions and begin to manage her diabetes. She felt back in control and like she had a say. Her circumstances hadn't changed at all. She still had gestational diabetes. Yet, now she felt like she was running the show, rather than the other way around.

As she continued to choose how to best manage diabetes, Leslie was examining and processing her emotions along the way. For example, each week after her doctor read her blood sugar results and decided to adjust her insulin level up, Leslie would start her self-coaching. She would tell herself that she was not failing, that she was not screwing up, even though it felt like it! She reminded herself that she was doing everything they told her to do. Her body was just not producing enough insulin. Simple as that. So if her body wasn't making the insulin it needed, insulin would need to be added. And if more and more needed to be added as her pregnancy progressed, then that was what was going to happen. No need to feel bad about it. It was something she had to tell herself constantly, since it felt like she was failing a test nearly weekly. Leslie kept her eye on the bigger picture and was hopeful and expectant that her diabetes would resolve itself post-pregnancy.

It's useful to be aware of and to accept what's going on in your body. And, at the next layer, to understand and allow for your feelings about what's going on in your body. If we try to pretend that we're not disappointed, frustrated, embarrassed, overwhelmed, etc., then we can't move past those emotions to a mindset where you can choose your focus and subsequently feel better.

Check In. How are you feeling about what's going on with your body?

How can you accept any feelings you might have about being at the mercy of your body?

## Feeling more vulnerable

Carrying another person around with us 24/7 can make us feel more vulnerable in situations we might be able to take in stride when we're simply functioning "for one."

When I was pregnant with my son, I was at Wrigley Field during a rare tornado warning. Wrigley is one of the oldest ballparks around, so the aisles are narrow and the spaces are small and cramped. It's also very popular and games are always sold out. On that particular day, the sirens began to blare and everyone was advised to move from their seats to the concession areas inside the stadium. As people started moving in different directions and in the crowded walkways, people got pushed around and bumped into. From time to time as I made my way out of the seating area, I panicked. My reaction to the situation was intensified, I believe, because I felt I had to make sure my unborn baby was okay. I was panicking on his behalf. I wanted people to see that I was pregnant, and to make way for me and him, for goodness sake! In the end, we were both fine and never in any real danger. If I hadn't been pregnant at the time, I don't think I would have felt so vulnerable.

Natalie commuted on a hectic city subway train every day. She enjoyed it. She was a well-put-together commuter, with her compact backpack that rested flush against her back. It was easy for her to weasel her way into a spot, wrap her arm around a post, and read a chapter of a book on the way to work. She loved the energy she experienced in the underbelly of her city twice a day.

That perspective altered significantly during her second trimester. She no longer enjoyed the hustling and jockeying of the commute. She found herself thinking, "Stop pushing and shoving!" She wondered why people couldn't just slow down and realize that there was more to life than a good seat on the train ride home from work! With her protruding belly, she was worried about people bumping into her baby. She wondered what would happen if there was an emergency and everyone tried to evacuate at once. She got pretty worked up about it and asked herself what she wanted to do about it.

Natalie realized that there wasn't anything she wanted to do differently. She didn't want to figure out a different way to commute to work. So, she simply tried to accept that her view of her daily train rides had changed. For a while, she was going to feel vulnerable in a situation that once made her feel energized. It was startling to her, yet also understandable. She told herself time and time again that it was fine and healthy to be concerned about the safety of her unborn baby. She slowly adjusted to her altered perspective.

At some point, all of us feel vulnerable when we are pregnant. Maybe it's when you find yourself in a crowd like Natalie and I did. Maybe it's at work when you fear people will assume you've become more of a family woman and less of a career woman. You might wonder how other moms are judging you as you sit in the doctor's office waiting for your appointment. There are often times that we feel *more* concerned or vulnerable in a situation simply because we are pregnant. And, it's useful to be aware of this.

Check In. In what situations do you feel more vulnerable because you're pregnant?

## Surrendering

A few months into my first pregnancy, I woke up in a mood. I quickly identified it as a hormone-induced mood. Wow, here it was. I felt totally out of control of my emotions. I was irritated and disappointed and no amount of rationalizing in my head or trying to distract myself could change it. I was stuck. I didn't feel like myself and didn't want anyone to realize that I had become that "crazy pregnant lady." I *so* didn't want to be her, but there I was feeling crazy and out of sorts. I had no idea what I was going to do.

The first time it happened, I did my best to stamp it down and to hide it. I fought myself all day long, hoping that it would go away. I hated myself and how I felt and how I was being that day. I nearly snapped my husband's head off that night. It was miserable.

I talked with my coach the next day, when I was feeling decidedly more like myself. Even though I was feeling better, I was so disappointed with myself and what I had experienced the previous day. I was beating myself up pretty good.

Knowing that hormonal days were bound to show up again and knowing that I didn't want a repeat of what I had just been through, my coach and I worked on different perspectives or approaches I could try. We brainstormed some possibilities: I could cancel all appointments on those days, in essence calling in sick. I could continue to do my best to mask it. I could keep it together for most people and just let my husband experience the wrath. As we were generating ideas, I didn't immediately see a "feel good" path.

Gradually, I began to see that I could actually surrender to the hormones. I could let the hormones win, choose not to fight them. Fighting them wasn't fun. It did not serve me to be in a battle all day long. What if I just gave up at the beginning of the day and said, "Okay hormones you win!"? I got excited about this.

"What would that look like?" my coach asked. It would look like me freely admitting to others that I saw or spoke with on "those" days that I was having a hormonal day. It was letting others know that I wasn't sure how I'd react to things that day. I might cancel some commitments if I wasn't in the emotional place to enjoy them. But, it was doing this without feeling guilty or wrong about it. It was bringing some humor to the experience. It was saying "Uncle" to my own chemical makeup.

My coach asked me how I could remember to do this the next time it occurred. I made a little white flag and I carried it around in my purse. It was my reminder to surrender, and it came in handy on more occasions than just those hormonal days. I know, yet often forget, that focusing on what we don't want gets us more of what we don't want. When we get anxiously engaged in wishing that something is *not* the way that it actually is, then we keep our focus on what we don't want. We get more evidence that things are *not* the way we want them to be. It's the difference between focusing on making a hormonal day go away and focusing on how to surrender to a hormonal day. It was also helpful for me to surrender when I needed to buy bigger pants and when people made (what I saw as) annoying comments to me.

A need to surrender may show up in a different area for you. Perhaps surrendering to the anxiety of going into an unpredictable delivery process will be important to you or accepting the fact that you're going to be pregnant on your birthday and need to alter your typical celebration. You are not in control of all that is happening. Yet, you can be in control of how you respond.

This is not to say that this idea of surrendering allowed me to completely rid myself of any moments of annoyance, disappointment, or resistance. There certainly were still plenty of those! And, I know, the times that I was able to surrender were transformative.

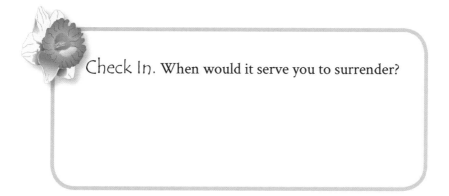

Check In. When would it serve you to surrender?

## Wanting the information you have to feel helpful

When we have in-depth knowledge about pregnancy or childbirth, it can be difficult to set that knowledge aside and simply have our own experience and allow our feelings to unfold naturally. It seems easy to take the knowledge we have and make assumptions about how we'll think and feel throughout the process.

Nurses, midwives, doctors, doulas, and other practitioners know about what needs to happen for a healthy baby to be born, and they have access to what can go wrong during a pregnancy. And, since pregnancy happens all the time, we *all* have some information, even if it's limited, about pregnancy and about what has happened with others. This information can leave us feeling discouraged about the inevitability of dealing with certain challenges, intensely focused on ensuring we don't experience certain outcomes, confident that we have the know-how we'll need, and/or assuming that we are going to feel certain ways. How do you let your knowledge and awareness empower you, rather than hinder you? How do you avoid assumptions that will keep you from experiencing your own authentic emotions?

Laura, as an educator in the area of prenatal parenting, had loads of information about pregnancy and embryology. I asked her about how this knowledge helped or hindered her during her own pregnancy. She confessed that she did often find herself, especially during the first trimester, feeling anxious about what she knew should be happening inside of her body. She thought through the details of what her body needed to manage. It got overwhelming at times, which was not what Laura had wanted to feel during her pregnancy.

She wanted to feel confident and peaceful about the life growing inside of her. So, she intentionally let herself forget everything that she knew about the development of the fetus in the womb. She didn't want to get into a consistent habit of instructing her body what to do: "Make the toes, remember there should be five. Now it's time to develop those lungs." She knew she couldn't micro-manage this process so she didn't want to feel like she was. Instead, she wanted to feel open and allowing and trusting. She wanted to let life work in her. Her approach, to step away from all the facts and data in her head, was successful. When she was pregnant, she felt confident that her body was working the way it needed to. She didn't apply the prenatal growth and development charts she had seen so often to herself, and she felt free and unencumbered as a result.

After having watched her friends go through pregnancy and having heard their complaints about their changing bodies, Erin assumed she'd have some major adjustments to make mentally about the weight she'd gain. She was actively telling herself that she didn't need to feel self-conscious, that the weight gain would be temporary, and that she didn't want to make herself miserable by obsessing about it. It seemed, in hindsight, that she had all these pep talks for no reason. As she progressed in her pregnancy, she didn't at all find herself concerned about the weight she was gaining. What she assumed would be a problem turned out to be a total non-issue.

Instead, Erin found herself being nagged by a much different kind of apprehension. It began to dawn on her that she was distressed about what kind of mom she'd be. She didn't consider herself very nurturing. And, the moms she saw around her seemed to be extremely maternal and nurturing. How was she going to pull this off?

It took a while for Erin to recognize this apprehension. Her focus had been so firmly on diminishing any worry about weight gain that she hadn't tuned into what else was going on.

Once Erin stopped masking her concerns and allowed her true apprehension about what type of mom she'd be to surface, she was able to process her thoughts and feelings about it. She realized there were many ways to "nurture" and that she wasn't going to naturally mimic the approaches of the moms in her community. She got excited about discovering her unique way of being a nurturing mom (now that she was no longer gearing herself up to handle a weight gain that wasn't negatively affecting her!).

Check In. How are you allowing the pregnancy information that you have to *help* you?

How are you allowing the pregnancy information that you have to *hinder* you?

## The perfection trap

Nichi was a doula. Every time she witnessed another woman's pregnancy or childbirth experience, she was busy creating an encyclopedia in her head. She'd think, "Note to self, don't let this happen. Make sure that you take care of yourself so you can avoid that." Since she assumed she'd be pregnant and give birth in the future, she knew she could apply what she was learning to herself one day.

When that day came, she had her encyclopedia of knowledge filed up in her head. She also had her strong belief that her attitude, her feelings, her thoughts, and what she ate would affect her baby and how she felt physically. She had seen positive and negative aspects of this phenomenon with the women she worked with. She wasn't being overly restrictive, but she did stay mindful of her thoughts, feelings, and actions and ensured that she was staying in the most empowering place she could.

Nichi marched off down the path of being in tune with her emotions and setting intentions for herself and her baby. She was enjoying much success. Those around her began to treat her as the poster child for how to do pregnancy and home birth "right." And in many ways her experience *was* poster-worthy.

Along the way, a nagging, overwhelming feeling crept up on her that everything had to be perfect and that *she* had to be perfect. Pressure was mounting because women were looking to her to be a great success story. What kind of message would it send if she – with her knowledge and commitment – couldn't have a great experience? She had to make sure she was on top of everything. She had to make sure it all went perfectly, otherwise what were these women going to learn from her? What had she learned about herself?

Tuning into her own feelings, Nichi saw the signs that she was getting nervous and was constantly fretting about doing everything "right." When she noticed this shift in her emotions, she had to remind herself that her job was simply to set her intentions and stay focused on what she and her baby wanted. Any belief that the process had to go a certain way or had to look a certain way were going to get in the way of Nichi having the peaceful, empowering experience she wanted. In time and with self-awareness, she was able to apply what she knew about pregnancy, and, at the same time, keep her expectations in check, reminding herself that she didn't fully know what to expect because she and her baby had never done this before. She couldn't control her outcomes, but she could set herself up for success.

Nichi's experience overall, although not "perfect," was certainly "poster-worthy." Most days she felt peaceful and grounded about the approaches she was taking. She worked and exercised until days before she delivered, keeping her body strong and fluid. And, in the end, Nichi delivered a 9 pound baby at home with no tearing, no hemorrhaging, and no problems.

Even if we're not like Nichi, with dozens of people watching our every move and expecting unending perfection, there are probably some elements of our pregnancy that we want to be "perfect." There is usually at least one thing that we desperately hope will work out just as we want. It may be a desire to not gain too much weight or to never have a hormonal outburst or to only eat healthy or to not have our pregnancy impact our ability to do our work, etc. We launch ourselves into a perfection pitfall if we feel it has to work out in a specific way… or else!

It's useful to identify our pregnancy perfection pitfalls. Chances are that we won't experience perfection. So if we're consciously or subconsciously striving for flawless, we're likely setting ourselves up for disappointment. We want to give ourselves some leeway, like Nichi did. When we identify our perfection pitfalls, we then can look at why this area is so important to us.

As an example, Heather was somebody who didn't want her pregnancy to impact her ability to do her work. She didn't want to *ever* have to tell a client or a business partner that she couldn't meet a deadline because she was overly tired or nauseous or distracted. To her, it seemed super wimpy. She wanted to be a person who was able to handle it all with ease and style. She saw – because of the rigidness of her thoughts and the tension in her body – that being "absolute" was a little crazy, so she looked at why it was so important to her. She was, at the end of the day, concerned about always being viewed as dependable and responsible, even when pregnant. She didn't want anyone to think she was making excuses.

Heather talked to one of her business partners about her feelings and her partner gently pointed out how hard Heather was being on herself. They went on to talk about how "stuff" comes up for everyone, that's life. Heather was able to lessen the expectations she placed on herself, and saw that, if she was so concerned about finishing things on time, she needed to create realistic timelines that would work for her. She built in extra time for pregnancy and life to happen. As you might guess, this inquiry represented a great "life" lesson as well as "pregnancy" lesson for Heather.

Check In. What are you trying to do perfectly?

Why is this important to you?

## Feeling needy

When we're pregnant we need things that we didn't previously need. It might be additional sleep, new clothes, understanding as we lift less or run out of a meeting to throw up, graciousness as our hormones cause us to get more emotional, help watching our older children – it might be a great many things. We're used to handling a lot in life, operating at a certain level and intensity. This may need to shift as we're pregnant or as we're in different periods of our pregnancy. As a result, we may be left feeling "needy." And, for many of us, feeling needy doesn't feel good. Neediness can leave us feeling weak, insecure, uneasy, pathetic, self-centered, or other emotions.

Mary Anne found herself wanting to ask for something that seemed really hard to ask for. It was difficult to ask because in doing so she felt she'd be succumbing to weakness and self-centeredness. Before she was pregnant, Mary Anne typically walked eight city blocks from the train station to her office building, enjoying the physical exertion and the idea that she was saving her family money by not taking a cab. While she was pregnant, she started to resent this walk that used to invigorate her. It took longer, she was getting sweaty, and she wanted to get to work earlier in the mornings to take care of things while she felt fresh and alert.

She wanted to talk to her husband about spending money on cab rides, and it was a hard conversation for Mary Anne to decide to initiate. She kept telling herself that she should toughen up, that it was good for her and the baby to get this exercise every morning. She thought about the weekly cost she'd incur and felt guilty and self-indulgent. Yet, the desire did not go away, and she finally broached the subject with her husband, sharing both her concerns and her guilt.

When her husband didn't immediately understand, Mary Anne admits she considered abandoning the request. But she pushed on. Even if he thought it was frivolous or unnecessary, she had finally given herself permission to feel how she felt and to want what she wanted. Once her husband understood the significance of the request, he was more than happy to agree to spend the money. Receiving the empathy and agreement from her husband helped Mary Anne further accept her desire as reasonable and not as an assessment that she was weak or needy.

Doreen felt that she had done a pretty fair job getting support during her pregnancies. Having two children, she was vividly aware that it took a village to raise children. That's why it came as such a disappointment toward the end of her third pregnancy when she suddenly felt so completely overwhelmed.

When Doreen realized that she was beyond needing a little help and needed a whole shift in responsibilities, she knew rationally she could ask her husband for a complete shift, right away. Yet, it felt so uncomfortable that she had let it get to that point without any preamble or warning.

She needed to tell her husband that she could no longer be the one who took the lead in most aspects of household management. Even though it felt uncomfortable and almost unreasonable, Doreen told her husband what she needed. She realized it would create more troubles not to.

Mary Anne and Doreen both took some useful actions. They did what they could to accept the idea that they needed something they didn't previously. And they acknowledged the feelings that went with that – the guilt, the overwhelm, the self-indulgence, the frustration, and the upset. Once they did that, then they were in a place where they could powerfully determine what they'd like to do. We all have that opportunity. Mary Anne and Doreen both had requests to make of their husbands. The actions we might choose to take could include just having someone listen, receiving some empathy, or asking for specific things we want and need.

Check in. In what ways are you feeling needy?

What do you want or need to help you accept and/or minimize this feeling?

## Embracing your feelings

Accepting our emotions during pregnancy, opening ourselves up, giving ourselves permission to make uncomfortable requests... This can feel like we are engaging in a lot of personal development work. Well, it is. Yet, it does not go without reward. There are some unbelievable benefits we can experience.

After weeks of trying to decide whether to approach her manager or not, Jasmine finally told her boss that she was having a hard time focusing during their staff meetings because they were held at 9:00 a.m., the time her morning sickness generally kicked in full force. Although worried that she'd appear weak and needy, Jasmine had come to the conclusion that she needed her boss to know what was going on and that any signs of being unfocused or not fully contributing to the discussion was based on something outside of her control. She was pleasantly surprised by the response she got. Not only was her boss empathetic, he was so glad she had told him. He hadn't been able to figure out why she hadn't had more to say about a few issues brought up at the staff meetings! He scheduled time to get her input separately and found a new time for the staff meeting that worked for everyone. Jasmine was glad she set her feelings of vulnerability aside and opened up to her boss.

Kira was part of a big family. Each Sunday she'd spend the majority of the day at her grandmother's house. When she was pregnant, Kira felt resentful that her family wouldn't let her do anything. They didn't want her to help with the meal or crawl around in the basement with the kids – nothing. Kira knew that they loved her and simply wanted her to take it easy, but it really frustrated her. She wanted to help. She wanted to truly spend time with her family, not sit in the corner by herself. She found them overbearing and patronizing, and didn't know how to ask them to change without hurting their feelings. She was frustrated and angry, yet also worried about broaching the subject with her family.

Eventually, instead of telling them about how she thought they were being – namely, demeaning and too protective – she decided to tell them more about what she wanted and what would make her feel best during her pregnancy. She told them the pregnancy was all about family for her and that she wanted to spend time doing things with all of them. Yes, she'd make sure to not overdo it, but she wanted to be in the kitchen and she wanted to watch the kids. She asked them to understand, and they did. It didn't stop them from asking her, "Are you sure you shouldn't take a break now?" and hovering over her at times. Yet that conversation, that had once seemed so impossible for Kira to broach, did get her out of the corner and interacting with her family again. Kira felt relieved and proud that she found an effective way to frame the conversation and share her feelings.

For Jasmine and Kira both, the first step was to be aware of how they were feeling. Then, they found a way to set their concerns aside, amid perceived judgments of others, to share how they were *really* feeling. They were authentic with themselves and with others. It was scary when they opened up to others. Still, they both believed that it felt better to let the feelings out, rather than to keep them in.

When we fully own, stop resisting, and admit to our feelings, we're able to release the hold they have on us. The emotions are no longer secretly in charge, running the show behind the scenes. We've brought the feelings out into the open where we can see them and deal with them and ultimately learn from them.

Check In. What feelings are you freely and fully embracing?

What feelings are you currently resisting?

## Learning from emotions

Processing feelings may seem like an overwhelming, never-ending activity during pregnancy. You're not going to get an argument from me! And, as I've already shared, I believe there is so much we can learn from the authentic processing of our emotions.

Tammy provided a great example of what's possible when we let our emotions in, experience them, and learn what they have to teach us. Tammy experienced a short pregnancy that ended in a miscarriage and a confusing, disappointing, and invasive process to remove leftover tissue. She was willing to share her story with me shortly after her post-miscarriage procedure and had a lot to say about what she was taking away from the experience.

The bottom-line is that Tammy learned a more effective way to deal with disappointment. After her miscarriage, she saw that when she felt hurt and confused, she tended to withdraw. She distanced herself from others by going into her "I'll just handle this all myself" mode, and she withdrew, to a degree, from her emotions by working to "handle" the situation, rather than just allowing herself to experience her feelings. She realized the detrimental consequences of her withdrawal. She felt all alone, misunderstood, and unsupported. Since she hadn't let anyone in, they didn't know how to help her.

She then intentionally reminded herself to communicate with her husband and others and to not retreat. She knew she wanted to process her feelings, rather than just power through her circumstances. By staying with it with her husband and sometimes talking when there didn't even seem to be a purpose to talking, Tammy felt more connected to her husband and saw her marriage strengthen. She learned she could simply allow her emotions to be what they were. She didn't have to apologize for them or pretend they weren't as intense or prevalent as they were. Being able to recognize and talk about her feelings helped loosen the negative hold they had on her. It didn't mean that the hurt and confusion quickly went away. Yet, it did mean that she no longer felt powerless or alone and solely responsible for figuring out how to deal with the disappointment and move forward.

By fully acknowledging her sadness and confusion, she couldn't ignore the fact that she needed a type of support and compassion, to help her through this period of disappointment, unlike any she had ever needed previously. Tammy learned to speak up for herself and set boundaries. She started pushing herself out of her comfort zone to ask for what she wanted or needed, even when she could tell that others didn't agree or understand why she was asking. She discovered approaches she could employ when life presented her with an obstacle, a difficult situation, and/or a disappointment. Because Tammy was willing to be guided by her emotions, she walked away from this experience with more than, "That sucked. I can't believe what I just went through." Yes, that time in her life did suck and yes, at times, she adamantly wishes she hadn't experienced it. And, she's learned lessons that will lighten her load and make a difference wherever her life may take her.

Even seemingly little, nagging emotions can teach us. Annie, for example, started feeling anxious at the end of her first trimester. She felt worried about her growing To Do list and guilty about not spending more time with her extended family. She just felt pressure nagging at her. As she let herself sit with and examine these feelings, she saw that she did a pretty bad job of taking care of herself on a day-to-day basis. Since she was good at getting frequent massages and taking regular vacations, she neglected to consider that she wasn't good at daily self-care. Her anxiety led her to this insight.

When she allowed herself to cut back on her volunteer hours and to take Saturday afternoons "off" from any household chores, she was surprised by how she felt. Instead of feeling irresponsible and worried about taking time away from the people and projects in her life, she felt even more responsible, empowered, and proud that she was taking great care of herself and her baby.

Our stories may be starkly different from Tammy's and Annie's, yet I think we all have the opportunity to learn lessons from our emotions. Uncomfortable or unwanted feelings let us know that it may be time to change our tactics, try something different. Feelings like those of joy, connectedness, and relief show us we're on the right track. These emotions let us know that we're finding "our" way.

What we learn from our feelings – the approaches we discover we want to employ – can be quite varied. In fact, in a situation where one woman might discover that she needs to reach out to people to best support herself, another may learn that giving herself some alone time is the best tactic. Additionally, the approach that works today, may not be as effective tomorrow. It's a continual learning process.

Whatever we're experiencing in pregnancy, there are emotions that come up that are designed to teach us. We can experience the negative emotions and feel badly that we're having them *or* we can experience the negative emotions and take away something positive.

Check In. What emotions – even if seemingly negative – have been gifts?

What have you learned?

## OKAY, LET'S BE REAL... ✿ ✿ ✿ ✿ ✿ ✿ ✿ ✿

Emotional shutdown needed!

Okay, let's be real. There are times when this "embrace your emotions and learn from them" sounds good in theory, but it just does not work in reality. When intense, uncomfortable, or unfamiliar feelings seem to be taking over, there are going to be times when you just don't have it in you to "embrace" them. Sometimes we just feel fed up or so over-the-top e-mo-tion-al about it all and completely incapable of processing any feelings in a practical, reasonable manner. A different course of action may be necessary...

Let yourself shutdown emotionally, if you need to. Throw your hands in the air and refuse to make any decisions! Sometimes simply waiting out the emotional onslaught is the best we can do. That's fine. Making significant decisions while we're experiencing an equally significant hormone fluctuation may not even be advisable.

There are times when we all might need to say "Screw you!" to personal growth and development and take an extended timeout. Feel free to take a hiatus from any enlightenment! The opportunities to learn and grow and develop will keep coming...you can be sure of that.

## Feeling bad about feeling bad

It's not always fun to deal with negative emotions. It sometimes may not even seem like the appropriate thing to do. Why spend more time on emotions that don't feel good in the first place? Why give them more attention? Why look them square in the face? Isn't that only going to make you feel worse?

If you have this assumption, you're not alone. There's a lot emphasis today about the power of positive thinking. And I agree that there is great value in this practice. Yet, at the same time, what we resist persists. If we resist looking at negative thoughts and concerns, they will stick around. Sweeping something unpleasant under the rug so we don't have to deal with it doesn't make it magically disappear. It just makes a little bump under our rug. The negative considerations may even fester and grow as we're trying to pretend that they don't exist or will just go away.

If we're straight with ourselves and put our disempowering notions in the forefront and examine them, we can process them and understand why we're experiencing them. Only then can we reframe our negative emotions or choose to do something empowering about them.

There's another reason to take a closer look at our disempowering feelings. Negative emotions can have a double whammy affect. We feel bad about the thing that's negative, and then we feel bad for feeling bad. Here's how it works: Let's say you're feeling embarrassed by how short of breath you are when you walk more than two blocks. The feeling of embarrassment is unpleasant, and then you take it a layer deeper and give yourself a hard time for feeling embarrassed, thinking something along the lines of, "I shouldn't care about being out of breath. I should embrace that as an aspect of the third trimester of my pregnancy!" You begin with the bad feeling of embarrassment, then you add a layer of feeling bad about the bad feeling. It happens all the time. We don't stop at the level of "Okay, I'm feeling embarrassed." We add another negative emotion on top of it. So, if we're able to deal with the feelings of embarrassment head on, we can avoid the phenomenon of building ourselves a little tower of negative emotions.

Toni, like many of us, struggled with weight gain during her pregnancy. She felt like she woke up one morning and all of a sudden her thighs were rubbing together and she had deep folds in her belly that she'd never had before. She felt big and sloppy and this frustrated her. Toni had been an athlete throughout her life. She knew her pre-pregnancy body well, knowing when to cut back or increase her food intake based on what sports she was involved in and how much she was physically exerting herself. She got mad at herself for seeming to forget this during her pregnancy. She was so annoyed that she hadn't gotten involved in sports or activities that would work well during a pregnancy and that she hadn't watched more closely what she'd been eating. Then, as she noticed this frustration and annoyance, she got mad at herself for feeling that way. Feeling frustrated wasn't going to improve her situation or get her moving in a more positive direction. She knew that and thought she was being so stupidly counter-productive. She was now annoyed with herself – and calling herself stupid – for being annoyed! Toni had gotten herself into a loop of feeling bad about feeling bad.

Toni soon realized that she was piling negative feelings on top of negative feelings. She could be annoyed about being annoyed…or, she could just let herself be annoyed. She could let that be her most prevalent emotion without judging it or saying it shouldn't be. Doing that allowed Toni to deal with her frustration in a straight-forward manner. She was able to look forward and make some changes to her schedule and eating habits, she was no longer angry at herself and feeling stupid about her emotional reaction. She was allowed to feel frustrated. It was a frustrating situation! And, it was actually from a place of frustration that she started doing what she knew to do and what she knew would work for her.

It is all too common for us women to lack compassion for ourselves. In order to fully accept uncomfortable feelings like disappointment, anger, or shame, we usually need to bring compassion into the equation. When we can be gentle and kind to ourselves, knowing that we're human, fallible beings, then we can actually let our initial layer of emotions in and let them serve their purpose, rather than piling a second layer of negative emotions on top. Toni could consider that her feelings of disappointment and anger were simply trying to tell her to make a change, not that she now needed to label herself as "stupid" as well.

Check In. Where are you feeling bad about feeling bad?

How can you stop?

## You've got what it takes

There is a lot about pregnancy that we have to look at and grapple with as expectant moms. There are all the physical changes we face and emotions that surface about the fact that we are pregnant. That's even before we consider what might be the most foundational shift in your world – that you are now a mother! Or, if you've been through pregnancy before, you're a mom to two kids or three kids, or more! You are now responsible for this yet-to-be-born baby. You are going to care for a newborn baby in a matter of months.

That can be a lot to take in and it can affect you in ways you don't expect or are not completely aware of. Changes to your lifestyle have begun already, and there are going to be more. It's a situation that's ripe for insecurities to come to the surface.

The questions I've asked myself or I've heard from other women are numerous: What if I'm not nurturing enough? If I can't manage my own schedule, how can I manage someone else's? How will I raise my kid – keeping him safe, not smothering him -- yet helping him develop into a self-sufficient independent adult? When my baby cries, will I know why? Will I know how to soothe her? Will I resent the loss of freedom in my schedule? How am I going to handle my heart and head being wrapped up in another person? Am I going to have to change as a person? Are there things I can no longer do now that I am a mom? Are there ways of thinking that I'll have to change? Am I mature enough for this? Am I selfless enough?

It's normal to have insecurities and wonder if you're doing the mom thing "right." However, you don't have to fit anyone else's mold of what a mom should be. Pregnancy is an opportunity to reflect and discover your own way. Know that you don't have to do what you see others doing.

Bridget realized that she had spent too much time and energy trying to determine if she and her baby were doing it right during her first pregnancy. She wanted to know all the numbers at her doctors' visits. How was her belly measuring? What was the estimated current weight of her baby? How did these compare with the norms? She asked all her friends who were moms about what they ate, how much they slept, what items needed to be on her baby registry, and more. She always felt good after she got answers that confirmed that she and her baby were "on track," yet she wondered why she worried in the first place. Why did she need this external validation? Why couldn't she trust that she and her baby were doing just fine?

The need for external validation continued for Bridget, even after her daughter was born. Bridget had learned that a nursing baby was supposed to feed on one breast for 10 or more minutes in order to get to the "hind" milk, the most valuable and nutritional milk. That made sense to her, but her daughter wouldn't eat for that long on one side. The milk would be gone and her daughter seemingly satisfied long before they reached 10 minutes. Many feedings consisted of only four minutes on each breast, although they took place at normal intervals throughout the day. The feedings just went super fast. Bridget made note to ask her lactation consultant and others about the short feedings.

That's when it occurred to Bridget that although the feedings were fast compared to what she was told was "normal," they didn't feel fast to Bridget. They felt normal. She suddenly wondered why she was going to pursue the question with the lactation consultant. She didn't need to talk to others. She realized that she felt peaceful and knew deep down that her baby was getting the milk and nutrition that she needed. Actually, it made her feel lucky. She got to experience the joys of breastfeeding in half the time! Her confidence that all was well was validated at her daughter's four-day-old doctor appointment when her daughter was already back to weighing more than her birth weight (babies typically lose a little bit of weight just after being born).

Bridget took on the idea that she could simply trust herself and her baby, and carried this notion with her into her next pregnancy. She didn't worry about what others were doing or what was typical, she simply looked for what seemed to work for her. It was a completely refreshing perspective for Bridget. When a question arose, she took a moment and tuned into her own intuition, rather than running around and asking others a bunch of questions. That realization she had when she was breastfeeding changed the way she approached motherhood and her next pregnancy. She felt much more grounded and self-assured.

Check In. What doubts do you have about being a mom?

What could help you release these doubts?

## One step at a time

The idea of motherhood can be overwhelming. Thinking about all the phases that you go through as a mom to growing children, it's easy to break out in a cold sweat! Remember that it's an evolution. Know that you get to make the journey one baby step at a time.

From your current position as a pregnant woman, motherhood can look overwhelming. From this view you're going to do so many new things such as deliver this baby (no small task), figure out how to best feed her and diaper her and put her to sleep (usually while family and friends look on), make choices about her care, help her expand and grow, keep her safe as she's learning to walk, encourage her independence, find the best disciplinary approaches, make choices about how much TV she can watch, worry about who she's friends with, be the one she counts on for everything, be the one she thinks is so lamely stupid, worry about peer pressure, do the best job you can instilling values, and let her make her own way in the world. It's a dynamic and ever-changing job and each child is different.

The emotions you'll experience along the way might resemble a roller coaster. There are likely to be ups and downs. It's likely that you're not going to feel confident, peaceful, and grounded all the time or about all aspects of motherhood. You'll be learning all the time. And, when you're not feeling as peaceful and assured as you'd like to be, that's the time to remind yourself that you are – in that moment – learning and expanding your capacities. Moms who have gone before you can tell you this: We don't do it perfectly, yet we now easily handle things that at one point seemed insurmountable.

When I first got pregnant, I couldn't imagine being able to handle everything. I figured I'd be less of a business owner, less of a household contributor, less of a wife, and generally someone who just couldn't get as much done as she used to. Yet, instead of being "less," I actually became "more." I've discovered that as an Entrepreneur, being a mom is not a limiting factor, it's a benefit. I have to be creative. I have to know my priorities. I no longer have time to muck around with the little, unimportant stuff. Being a mom has enabled me to improve my prioritization, time management skills, and ability to be present in the moment in ways I didn't think were possible before I had kids.

I also know I can be most effective when I use my emotions as a guide. Positive emotions such as excitement, momentum, pride, and confidence let me know that I'm organizing myself in ways that feel best to me. When I experience anxiousness, confusion, frustration, or overwhelm then I can look at what adjustments I need to make to shift myself into more positive emotions.

Check In. Where do you feel that you won't "live up" as a mom?

How can you reframe your thoughts and feelings?

By all accounts, it seemed that Carrie was breezing through motherhood. She had two kids and she made it look easy. She enjoyed being pregnant and adjusted fairly easily to shifting her time and energy to her kids. It was, after all, always what she wanted to do. She cut back on the hours that she worked as a nurse, and the hospital that employed her was happy with the arrangement. She felt competent and proud. She and her husband both wanted a lot of kids and they were well on their way to creating the big family of their dreams. Life was humming along.

When Carrie got pregnant with her third child, a little sooner than expected, she suddenly felt like a rug had been pulled out from underneath her and she didn't understand why. Why was she feeling unsettled about being pregnant with a third child when she and her husband had talked of having five? Why did preparing for this child feel so completely overwhelming? Questions that had never bothered her in the past now plagued her: Would she have enough time and attention for each of her kids? How was she going to balance it all? What kind of schedule could they work out so she could still work a shift or two a week? What would her days look like? Did they have enough room in the house? She was questioning things she had never doubted before.

At first, Carrie simply tried to ignore her doubts. These thoughts and feelings were so different from any she'd had in the past, she thought she should chalk them up to being overtired or having a strange surge of hormones at the start of her pregnancy. She tried to keep marching forward, ignoring the concerns. It didn't work. The questions kept cycling through her head, making her feel like she was on a train that was moving too fast.

Finally, she admitted to herself and to her husband that she was feeling anxious and overwhelmed about adding to their family again so soon.

It was hard. She liked feeling like the woman who was born to be a mom. She loved it when others said she made it look easy. Now here she was saying that it felt hard and that she was panicked.

Her husband said her anxiety was completely understandable, and Carrie felt a sense of relief begin to crack open as he said it. She didn't know how he'd handle her anxiety, since it had never been part of their reality before. He began to point out all the things that Carrie handled as a mother of two: how she managed four different schedules, crawled after a toddler when she was nine months pregnant, completely reorganized the office and storage space to make room for their second child. He reminded her that she instinctively knew what each kid needed, that she did a great job of taking care of herself during pregnancy, and more. Carrie was floored. Her husband had complimented her mothering abilities before, but she had been so busy taking it for granted (and doing what she needed to do) that she never really fully "saw" all she had handled. She let it in. In fact, when she looked at her role in all the ways their lives had shifted over the previous three years, she was amazed.

Her anxiety about having a third baby so soon did not magically melt away. Yet, acknowledging what she'd already handled so well helped Carrie to feel confident and determined to expand her capacities. She saw what a disservice she had done herself by brushing away others' compliments. She was a great, incredible, multi-tasking mom. And when people told her so, instead of dismissing their compliments she now thinks, "Yeah, I know!"

For all of us, it is important that we acknowledge what we do well. Sure, we feel like there's always going to be more we can do or something that we can do better. Let's not place our focus there. Instead, take time to feel great about all you accomplished. Every moment of every day, as an expectant mom, you're accomplishing something. Whether you're resting or getting yourself to the doctor or eating a snack or handling an irate client at work...(the list goes on and on), you deserve acknowledgement.

Check In. What are you doing well as an expectant mom?

## Embracing Your Feelings ✿ ✿ ✿ ✿ ✿ ✿ ✿ ✿ ✿

There are a range of new, strange, and sometimes unsettling or upsetting emotions that can come up for us during pregnancy. We have the opportunity to embrace these feelings and allow them to be an important guide for us. Our emotions can help us discover what choices are best aligned with our values and how we want to be and act as an expectant mom.

* Do what you can to fully let in the emotions you feel. From the highest of the highs to the most unsettling of the lows, all your feelings have lessons to offer you.

* Pregnancy helps you learn that you are not solely in control of what happens. However, you are in control of how you respond to what happens.

* It's easy to make assumptions about how you'll think and feel during pregnancy. Tune into your feelings and allow them to unfold naturally and authentically.

* Identify your pregnancy perfection pitfall – the aspect of pregnancy you desperately want to go perfectly – and find a way to reframe your expectations. Perfection pitfalls invite disappointment.

* It's beneficial to admit your true feelings to yourself and to others. Hiding from unwanted feelings may only make them grow and fester.

* When you share with others what is really going on, they are able to empathize and support you in a way that they couldn't otherwise.

* When you don't accept the "bad" feelings you feel, then you can find yourself feeling bad about feeling bad.

* It's important to acknowledge what you are doing well as an expectant mom.

Check In. What, for you, is most important to remember as you process your emotions?

# Choosing Your Care and Support

I think it's an important concept that we get to *choose* the care and support that will sustain us during our pregnancies. And by "care and support," I'm referring to everything from our professional care providers to day-to-day help to nourishing activities such as massages to emotional support and encouragement. We get to choose what works best for us in all of these scenarios; we are not stuck with what we get. We can ask. We can create. And, perhaps most importantly, we can freely accept what is offered to us. Often, as women, we're used to being the caretakers and don't do the best job of being cared for.

I encourage you to stretch yourself in this area. Continually look at how you can care for yourself, support yourself, and ask others to do the same for you. This means being engaged with questions such as:

* What do I want to do for myself?

* How can I ask others to help me?

* Who is the most supportive of me and my desires, and how can I spend more time with these people?

- ✤ Who would have good ideas for me about how to best handle this situation?

- ✤ What truly nourishes me and refuels me?

- ✤ Where do I feel stressed or trapped and what would help me release these feelings?

- ✤ What would feel luxurious?

- ✤ What would help me in this moment, right now?

- ✤ What are the characteristics of my ideal care providers?

- ✤ What kind of relationship do I want to have with my doctor or midwife or other practitioners?

- ✤ How can I give myself permission to unapologetically and unabashedly ask for what I need and want?

It's easy to get into the limiting thinking that you've got to make do with what's available or that your choices are limited to what is typical in a situation. Don't assume that you've got to go with the care provided at the hospital that your doctor typically uses, or that you shouldn't need or request something at work that other pregnant employees haven't asked for. You can always ask. Others can always say "no;" but that doesn't mean you can't ask.

I want pregnant women to set aside whatever apprehensions keep them from asking for what would best support them. (Personally, my worries were about appearing too wimpy or too high maintenance.) Often, if we ask others in a straight-forward manner, without laying down a guilt track, and truly give them the opportunity to say yes or no, we will find the assistance and encouragement we want and need. And, if we don't, we're still no worse off. In fact, the act of making a support request helps us clarify what would really help us. And once we know, we can look for other ways to receive the help.

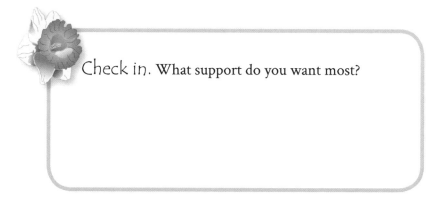

Check in. What support do you want most?

Let's hear about how different women enabled others to support and care for them while they were pregnant.

## Creating a support team

For her second pregnancy, Christi intentionally looked at a number of aspects of her life and hand-selected a team of people to support her. She had some unresolved issues about what occurred when she had her first baby – an unplanned pregnancy that resulted in an emergency c-section – and did not want to bring resentments and insecurities into her second pregnancy.

Even before she got pregnant, she was aware that she desperately wanted to avoid the experiences of her first pregnancy. Christi felt she had to figure it all out herself and determine all the information and techniques she needed in order stay empowered and peaceful. She put a lot of pressure on herself, until she realized that the pressure was neither empowering nor peaceful! Her idea of building a knowledgeable "dream team" to support her immediately took the pressure off. She knew she had found the approach that would work for her.

First, she clearly knew she wanted a midwife, and had specific requirements for that person. Christi desired a midwife who was easily accessible at any time of day for questions. She met with a number of perfectly lovely midwives, yet if they didn't indicate that they were set up for their patients to be able to contact them at any hour, Christi moved on.

Next, Christi was deliberate about spending time with those of her friends with whom she felt she could be "real" about what was going on, without having to sugar-coat or cast things in the best possible light. She allowed herself to lean heavily on these friends. They were the ones who helped her process out loud the disappointments around feeling like she didn't enjoy her last pregnancy and believing that she didn't advocate for herself as much as she should have during her delivery.

Christi worked as a healing professional, someone who works with a person's energy in ways to enable a body's own natural healing ability, so she knew what she was looking for in the healing professional she'd hire while she was pregnant. She took her time and met with a few until she was certain the individual possessed the characteristics and techniques she wanted. She also made the decision to take a sabbatical from her own work as a healing professional while she was pregnant. She knew it would serve her best to put her focus on healing and nurturing herself, rather than handling the sometimes emotional toll it takes to support others to heal.

Christi was delighted that she had a support team that was specifically and intentionally selected. In the past, she was often the go-to person for others. By building her team, she took that responsibility off herself and had her own go-to people. She loved the idea that she didn't need to know everything herself. She simply needed to know who to ask. This was a huge relief to Christi, and a complete shift from what she had been thinking just months before.

This is a great reminder for all of us. We don't have to know it all or do it all…if we don't want to. Each of us can create our own version of a support team that reflects our specific needs and areas of focus. Consider for a moment who could best assist and encourage you? Maybe you're seeking individuals who can calm you. Maybe it's someone who can get you riled up and excited. Maybe you want a masseuse, doula, reiki practitioner, acupuncturist, workout buddy, great listener, a doctor with a certain type of experience, a midwife with a specific kind of approach, friends who will tell it like it is, people who encourage you to think about yourself, and/or great brainstormers. It's up to you to determine what you want and invite people to play the perfect role for you.

Check In. Who would you like to have on your support team and how can each member best support you?

## A co-parent from the very beginning

Stacey was clear from the beginning of her pregnancy that having her husband, Steve, be a co-parent and equal partner right from the start would best serve her, her baby, and her family.

It's easy to think that Dad can't possibly be an equal partner during pregnancy because he's, well, not pregnant. Yet, Stacey knew she was going to want and need Steve to act as a true co-parent throughout their kids' lives. She felt the best way to achieve this was to create it right from conception. She was intentional about partnering with him and including him every step of the way.

When there was a doctor's appointment, it wasn't about what questions *Stacey* had for the doctor; it was about what questions *Stacey and Steve* had for the doctor. It also meant, at times, that Stacey had to reach out to her husband in ways that didn't feel natural. She often had to initiate and do most of the talking, especially when she was sharing what it was like to experience hormone fluctuations, to have your belly expand, to not be able to fit into "regular" pants anymore, and to feel so physically and emotionally connected to their baby.

There were also instances when Steve's paternal instinct kicked in and he took the lead. He researched childbirth classes, how and where to create a gift registry, and what type of stroller to buy. He got the car seats installed. He also logged hours in online discussion groups reading how other women dealt with the physical and emotional shifts that Stacey was experiencing. She was often surprised by what he had to bring to their conversations.

By taking the extra effort to share with and include her husband, Stacey had the glorious experience throughout her pregnancy of knowing that someone always had her back. She wanted and needed someone to lean on, someone to whom she could say, "I trust you with my life." There were times when Stacey would think she couldn't deal with the strain of the circumstances, and Steve was there for her, understanding who she was, what she was experiencing, and knowing that she could do it. And because they had been on the journey together, Stacey could believe Steve when he said, "You can do this. I know what you're made of."

There is a very practical aspect to including your partner in all aspects of pregnancy and relating to them as an equal partner in the process. It might not be easy to do since you are the one carrying around extra weight and physically nurturing two bodies for nine months. Yet, by relating to your significant other as your teammate from the beginning – from conception – it gives your mate the opportunity to grow into the role of co-parent.

Check In. How do you want to include your partner in the experience of pregnancy?

What difference would it make if you related to your non-pregnant partner as your true partner from the very beginning?

## Finding supporters and avoiding others

As she was contemplating getting pregnant and at the beginning of her pregnancy, Leslie carefully paid attention to who seemed most supportive of the choices she was making and who did not.

In general, Leslie tended to be open and often asked a lot of people their opinions. She used this approach when she considered adding to her family as a 44 year-old, recently divorced, single mom. She asked others her most pressing questions: How will this affect my baby as she grows up? What about impacts on the overall family? What about the baby's sibling? (Leslie had a 7-year-old daughter at the time.) She talked to a variety of people she knew personally and professionally. She wanted people to bring things to her attention that she wouldn't think of on her own. And she wanted to see which ideas and pieces of advice most resonated with her beliefs. She thought this was a very important process for herself in feeling grounded and at peace with her decisions. A terrific byproduct of the process was that she got a good sense of exactly where – with what people – she had her biggest support. She saw who got nervous and itchy when she brought up the topic. She saw who readily jumped into seeing possibilities and sharing ideas. She got clear about who she would and would not lean on heavily throughout her journey.

She didn't judge those who weren't immediately in agreement with her choice. She knew that having another baby at this time could look risky to others. She understood that and didn't try to convince any non-enthusiasts otherwise. She also knew not to seek them out at those times when she needed some encouragement.

Leslie's approach makes great sense. She didn't have to waste time trying to change another person's view and she still got the support she wanted and needed. So often, it's hard to simply let different perspectives be different. It's hard to not judge the other perspective – and other person – as "wrong." Readily accepting others' perspectives can be a transformative self-care act. Instead of trying to influence or change another person's view, we could simply just spend more time with those who have opinions or outlooks that best support us.

Check in. Where does your best support come from?

Where are you trying to get support, without success? Could you stop?

## Working it out at work

A special area of consideration for many women is how to handle their pregnancies at work. On the job, it's not always possible to simply spend less time with people who have what we consider "unsupportive" perspectives. Or we may have relationships that feel mostly "professional" and it feels awkward to discuss "personal" needs and the support we want.

Jen – someone who did an amazing job of intentionally choosing her doula and midwife and asked her husband and friends for support throughout her pregnancy – admitted that there was probably support available at work that she didn't seek out or ask for. Somehow work seemed to her like an area of life where she just needed to figure it out and make it work on her own. And figure out some creative strategies she did! For example, when her body told her, unequivocally, that it was time to sleep, she took naps under desks in empty offices.

Her figure-it-out-on-your-own mentality grew out of habits she created in her first trimester when she wasn't telling anyone she was pregnant. She didn't ask for what she needed then because her co-workers weren't aware of her circumstances. As her pregnancy progressed, the pattern of not asking for support continued. She told me that if she were to do it again, she would be more upfront with what she needed, even though it would take more audacity for her to ask for help at work than it did in other areas of life. Yet, she also acknowledged that you don't know what's available unless you ask!

Check in with yourself. What do you need to make work work for you? Our jobs are an area of life where we might spend the most conscious effort determining and demonstrating the kind of worker, contributor, employee we want to be. So, it may take the most intentional thinking to determine how you want to balance your personal needs and requests with your professional philosophies. It may help to bounce around ideas with someone else: perhaps a coach, a business mentor, or other working moms.

Check In. What ideas do you have to best work it out at work?

Some women have asked for *lots* of support from their husbands and families so they wouldn't need to ask for much at work. Amanda was a traveling, high-producing salesperson. She didn't see a way to significantly cut back at work or ask for support and still be the contributor she wanted to be. She allowed herself to get plenty of rest on the weekends. That meant asking her husband to do the grocery shopping, pick up around the house, and manage their social schedule – all things that Amanda used to handle. It even meant that her husband went to family functions without her on occasion. He agreed to do this because Amanda shared with him how much it meant to her to continue to excel at work while she was pregnant. She knew what a difference it made to her clients and to her co-workers when she put in the time and did a great job. And, she personally gained an important sense of accomplishment and pride in doing her work well and being the best salesperson in her company. Knowing she'd be taking maternity leave, and thinking there would be support she'd want to request once her baby was born, she was committed to taking the time before the baby came to get herself, her clients, and her co-workers set up as best she could.

That's what felt good for Amanda. It worked for her because she was straight with herself. She wanted to continue to operate in a certain fashion at work and was willing to ask for support and let go of expectations for herself in other areas of life to make that happen. It also worked because she made specific requests of her husband to support her. Amanda's choices were successful for her and her family.

Other women have found different solutions. Beth had her own business. As a solopreneur, she knew it would be easy to get caught up in thinking she had to do it all, including checking in with clients in the weeks immediately after her baby was born. It was what she thought she "should" do, but it wasn't what she wanted. She wanted to shut down her business completely for eight weeks and wanted to be able to work part-time for a space of time before and after her eight-week leave. So, after the first trimester, Beth told her clients and business partners about the leave she planned to take when her baby was born and the options they'd have in her absence. Clients could choose to take a break during her leave, work with someone else (with whom Beth would overlap services to ensure consistency), or change the schedule of their work to accommodate Beth's leave. Beth had thought it through as best she could and was confident that it could all be worked out. Her clients picked up on this confidence and everything did indeed work out easily.

Beth did some creative things she'd never done before. For example, she was scheduled to co-facilitate a workshop about a week-and-a-half before her due date. She decided to pay someone whom she and her co-facilitator trusted to be on "stand by" that day just in case she went into labor early. Beth negotiated one rate for the facilitator to prepare and be on standby and another should this person actually need to facilitate. It turned out that Beth was able to lead the workshop as planned. Still, she says it was money well spent to have a backup if she needed it. She wasn't comfortable just "hoping" she wouldn't go into labor prior to the workshop and leave her client and co-presenter high and dry. She got out in front of it and made sure things were taken care of.

Women in corporations (like Jen who I mentioned earlier) speak to the fears around asking for support in environments where people are working long hours, are relying on you to contribute to team projects, and/or are vying for the same promotion you want. It can feel scary and even self-sabotaging to ask for support during your pregnancy. You might not want to seem like you need "special" help or draw unwanted attention to any sort of perceived "lack." Christine battled this by reminding herself that we're all human and we all need something at some time or another. You may need help during your pregnancy. The next person might need help when his father gets sick. Another may need help when she gets a flat tire on the way to a big client presentation.

You can provide a great gift by accepting your vulnerability and asking for support. This can even open up the doors to your teammates doing the same. Since her pregnancy, Jen has seen this phenomenon take place at her office. As expectant and breastfeeding moms have asked for various things that would support them, others have felt encouraged to ask for what they need. The co-workers of these moms are grateful for the increased support they've received.

You know your work culture and commitments better than anyone else. You know what you're comfortable asking for and what you're not. I will tell you this, it's a common theme among women that I've interviewed who work in corporations to say that they wish they had asked for more. To quote Wendy, "Tell pregnant women they can ask for more than they think they can! Tell them it will be okay." Stretch yourself to do what will serve you best. And, trust yourself.

Check In. What support would you like at work that you're hesitant to ask for?

## ❀ OKAY, LET'S BE REAL… ❀ ❀ ❀ ❀ ❀ ❀ ❀ ❀ ❀

I don't want your so-called "help!"

A key theme of this chapter is to stretch yourself and create, request, and accept care and support. At the same time, let's be real and acknowledge there are some offers of help you don't want, or that don't feel supportive at all!

Some days, you simply don't want help…period.

Sometimes what is offered under the guise of "help" feels much more like meddling, than any kind of "helping."

Other times, you know exactly how you want to handle the situation and you don't want anyone to mess with or mess up your plan!

Whatever the reason, there will be times when the most "helpful" thing is to not receive any help. And you can let others know that. Simply decline their offers. Say "No" or "Not today." Get the person out of your business as soon as you can, if that is what will best support you in that moment.

It'd be nice if people would ask you what would be helpful, listen carefully to your response, and then provide it! It doesn't always work that way. There are times you're going to need to put your foot down and refuse.

Remember you can decline whenever the help offered is not actually helpful to you.

# Now is the time…

Taking great care of yourself and asking for support are really nice capacities to develop while you're pregnant. After your child is born and as he's growing, you'll be called upon to tend for him in new and ever-changing ways. If we all could learn in pregnancy to treat ourselves really well, then we'd help ourselves not fall into the trap of always putting ourselves last. And, when we're well-rested, fulfilled, and adequately nourished (and I'm not just talking about food), we are in the best position to take care of others. It's not a selfish act to get the care and support we want and need. Being well-cared for enables us to be there for others.

Tricia hadn't realized how much her seemingly selfish request was going to benefit her and her family. When she was pregnant with her second baby, Tricia's husband was traveling for work most of each week and she found herself overly tired and frustrated taking care of her toddler son and the household on her own. She felt like she had no time for herself. She got annoyed enough with the situation that she forced herself to ask her in-laws if they would watch her son one night a week.

This felt like such an audacious request to Tricia. She thought she should've been able to tend to her family all on her own. Yet, a voice was telling her that she had to find a way to get some time for herself. So, she asked. And they accepted!

At first Tricia used these evenings to vacuum, dust, prepare meals, grocery shop, and other things that are easier to do without a toddler underfoot. Then, she started sprinkling in dinners with girlfriends, an occasional massage, leisurely walks around the neighborhood, and curling up with a good book. She shifted from scurrying around trying to check as many things off her list as she could in this time, to treasuring the slowed-down time with herself. It became an opportunity to reconnect with who she was and what she enjoyed. She felt refueled after these evenings.

Much to her delight, her family enjoyed the new arrangement as well. The bond that grew between grandson and grandparents during Tricia's pregnancy was one that positively altered their relationships going forward. Her son knew that Wednesdays were "Granny and Papa" days. He appreciated Granny's cookies and learned new vocabulary as he and Papa "worked" on cars together. Tricia could see that her in-laws had a new appreciation for what it was like for her to care for her son by herself during the week while her husband traveled.

Tricia learned a valuable lesson during her second pregnancy: Asking for help can create a win/win/win situation for everyone! We have to remind ourselves that others might also benefit when we ask them to support us.

Taking good care of yourself during pregnancy gets you into the habit of practicing self-care, which will be useful for you in your ongoing role of "mom." I know that I want to be a role model of good self-care for my kids. I want them to see Mommy as a person with unique interests who has activities she enjoys that do, at times, take her away from her spending time with them. I want them to know that we all have the right to ask for what we want, to put ourselves first at times, and to have independent pursuits.

When I put self-care into this perspective - a framework of what I want for my kids - I clearly see what I can do to be a role model. I also believe our kids start learning from us in vitro. For multiple reasons, now's the time to intentionally tune into and create what would best support and care for you.

Check in. What stops you from engaging in the activities that would best support you?

How can you give yourself permission to fully care for yourself?

Even when you know theoretically that it can benefit everyone involved when you ask for assistance, it's still easy to forget it. In the moment, you might think of the act of asking for support as a weak one. Yet, remember this: it's a sign of strength, a sign that you are secure enough to admit when you don't want to or can't handle it all on your own, and a sign that you're gracious enough to let others contribute. So, remind yourself that asking for support is a reflection of inner courage and generosity, and do all that you can to give yourself permission to ask for help!

## What nourishes you?

Care and support can take many forms. One aspect, as we've discussed, is asking for help in specific situations like assistance with the housework or rearranging your work schedule.

But that's just the beginning. We also should consider what will truly *nourish* us. What could you do for yourself for no other reason than to simply be nice to yourself? What could you do that would go beyond getting "help" to getting indulgently "nourished"?

When you nourish yourself you refuel and energize yourself. Again, it's beneficial to you and those around you. When you engage in something that leaves you feeling good, you bring that good feeling to other areas of your life. Positive feelings and good choices lead to more positive feelings and good choices. So, what are some activities, hobbies, or interests in which you could engage that would have you feeling great?

There are some traditional nourishing activities that can come to mind like massages, hot baths, walks in the park, and time with girlfriends. These are great and a great start to the inquiry.

Think beyond these initial ideas. What else, specifically, could nourish *you*? Would it be nourishing to get more sleep? Do you want to change up how you spend your time? For example, I made a deal with myself in my third trimester that I wouldn't have more than two evening commitments per week and there'd be at least one day a week that I could sleep in.

Perhaps there are things you want to add to your schedule. Is it time for a pottery class, regular aerobics, or evenings alone in a coffee shop? What activities will best support you to feel relaxed, grounded, peaceful, energized, however you most want to feel? There are an infinite number of possibilities.

Check In. How do you want to nourish yourself and care for yourself during your pregnancy? (Be sure to include some ideas that stretch yourself. Think about what you want, not what you can easily get...)

Okay, some of you might be thinking that this "nourishment" idea is a good one in theory, yet not very doable in reality. You may question how you'd have the time or money to nourish yourself in any meaningful way. Perhaps you think nourishment is just a luxury that you can't afford. I hear you. I've had similar thoughts like, "I'm barely getting done what I need to, how am I going to do 'extra' activities? We've got a baby on the way, I need to be saving money for him or her!"

Remind yourself of a couple concepts. First, you will be better able to do all the things you need to do if you've refueled or renewed yourself in some way. Next, nourishing activities don't have to cost much or anything at all. A walk, a moment to listen to a favorite song, a chat with a friend all can be nourishing without breaking your budget or taking a lot of time.

## "Little" nourishments have big payoffs

During her pregnancy, Jen found herself getting into a mindset that she didn't have time for anything other than sleep! Her eyes would just begin to close of their own accord about 8:30 p.m., regardless of where she was or what she was doing. So, she started making sure she got herself to bed by that time. That was great and useful, yet it left her feeling like all she did was rush through her days so that she'd complete her commitments by the time her body started shutting down. She knew she was taking care of herself, but she also felt something was missing: fun, peacefulness, something. But how could she add even more to a day that was already overstuffed and shortened by her need for sleep? The key for Jen was reframing the question. It wasn't "How can I add in even more things to do every day?" it was "What could I do for myself, even if it was only for five minutes?"

She found many answers to the question. She could stop what she was doing, close her eyes, and take a few deep breaths. She set an hourly alert on her computer. When it went off, it was her cue to get up and walk around the office, giving herself a break and allowing herself to acknowledge all that she'd accomplished in the past hour. This practice of reflecting hourly turned out to be transformative for Jen.

She saw that some of the tasks she considered "must dos" really weren't. By eliminating non-essentials, she created more time and space for lunches with co-workers, walks outside after work, her new moms group meetings, and she still got herself to bed by 8:30 p.m. most of the time!

Jen took a few important, nourishing actions. She listened to her body and didn't resist this idea that she needed more sleep. She got clear that she wanted more nourishment. Even when she didn't initially see a solution, she didn't give up and kept searching for little ways to nourish herself. She identified short and simple ways to care for herself and she stuck with them. She enjoyed and capitalized on the insights her reflection time provided her!

Check in. What could you do to nourish yourself that would only take a few minutes each day?

What are your "must dos"? What would happen if you didn't do them?

There are small actions we can take to care for and support ourselves each day. There are other people that we can call upon to help us with those actions or to complete them for us.

We can also be intentional about how we interact with all the information, advice, and resources about pregnancy that are readily accessible these days. And, allow ourselves to do so in a way that feels empowering and comforting to us.

## What information do you want and need?

There is an endless supply of information about pregnancy available from friends and family, from books and the internet, even in TV and movies. How much information about pregnancy, what happens, and what might happen do you feel will be most supportive to you? Being clear about what you want to know and what you do not want to know can help you create the pregnancy experience you want.

Again, the spectrum here is incredibly wide. Some women want to read all the books and search the internet to understand every single thing they might be in for. The knowledge soothes them, even the seemingly "bad" news about ailments they might experience. That information is empowering because it makes them feel forewarned and prepared.

Others prefer to skim the available information, just getting a sense of what might happen and what resources might be most helpful if those things happen. They like knowing there are places they can turn, and they enjoy feeling informed, but in small doses.

Others don't want to know any more than they need to. They avoid reading pregnancy books focused on all the things that could go wrong during a pregnancy, and they'd prefer to not get worked up about something that might not even happen to them and create concerns where there weren't any before.

Check In. What's your overall approach to having or getting information about pregnancy and childbirth?

Knowing how much data you want to expose yourself to is one question that is helpful to answer for yourself. Understanding the amount and type of information you want in order to confidently make decisions regarding your care and support is another.

## What's an "informed" decision?

The preferred amount and type of information needed to make what feels like an "informed" choice can vary greatly from one woman to another. Some women feel best after doing a certain amount of overall due diligence, other women rely more heavily on intuition, others limit themselves to a few pieces of key information, and others trust they'll know it when they see it.

The question about how much information you need in order to feel confident in your decisions regarding your care is an interesting one. It's something that's useful to consider even before you start to gather information about possible choices such as when to get prenatal massages, what kind of body pillow you might want, whether you want to hire a doula, and/or if you want to invite your mom into your delivery room. When you have clarity about how much is enough, you don't have to gather more information than you need. You can also let the choices be easy. It could be that someone makes a suggestion, you feel your energy and intuition line up with it, and it's done. You don't have to create a full-blown research project – unless a full-blown research project is the way that feels best for you. Like your choices, your method of choosing is yours to declare.

I would suggest understanding clearly where you land on the continuum from painstakingly over-deliberation to not giving a decision one iota of thought. Somewhere in between those extremes is your perfect balance. It's useful to know which direction you tend to favor and, at times, to play the friendly devil's advocate with yourself.

If you're one who tends to rigorously complete a vast amount of due diligence, you can ask yourself: "Why am I getting this information? Will this type of information actually impact my decision? What do I really need to know?" If you tend to resist research at all costs, you can ask yourself: "Is there information I'd like to have to confirm my choice or that would help me make a confident choice? What questions do I have that I'd like to get answered?"

Remember that "research" can take many forms: from talking to people about their choices and preferences, to looking online, to reading books, to talking to experts, to personal trial and error. Additionally, the kind of information that speaks most clearly to you and what feels inconsequential varies from person to person. There isn't a right way or a wrong way. Trust what has you feeling confident and peaceful.

Check In. How much information and what type of information do you need to confidently make choices regarding your care and support?

I tend to be someone who plays on the "I don't like research, let's not do that" side of the continuum. While working on this book, I found myself questioning whether that approach was the "right" one. Someone's comment during an interview completely rattled me and caused me to question how I chose where to deliver my baby.

I interviewed Sarah, who had a business supporting women to make well-informed decisions about their pregnancy and delivery care options. As a result, she was quite knowledgeable about resources and options in my area. I was pregnant at the time and as she and I conversed after her interview, she asked me about what hospital I was going to and who my doctor was.

When Sarah shared that my hospital was not one she'd recommend, it left me doubting myself, and I didn't want to feel that way. All I could say to her was that I was disappointed she said that to me. The conversation ended awkwardly and uncomfortably.

Again, Sarah was passionate about getting women all the information there is to know about their choices. This is an important service because there are women who want this level of information to feel comfortable that they've made a well-informed decision.

As I spoke to Sarah, my initial reaction was to feel irresponsible about not doing extensive research on choices in my pregnancy and my life. But when I really looked, I saw that I didn't actually believe I was irresponsible. When I see people investigating three different tuxedo shops while planning their wedding, I think it's a colossal waste of time. And, I feel, data can be construed different ways. (Not knocking you data-junkies, I've spoken to a lot of you and you are able to get to a place of grounded, unshakeable confidence about your choices using it. It's inspiring.) What became clear to me after our conversation was that I do not have the same approach, nor do I personally value that level of detail. The data I rely on is different than statistics and percentages. I rely more on experience and intuition.

My interaction with Sarah, although it didn't initially feel good, was a huge blessing. It helped me get clear on my natural decision-making process. It allowed me to accept that there were many different "responsible" decision-making approaches, including my own! It also helped me get to a place where I felt really good and at peace about my hospital choice.

It's easy to think that women who do not make important decisions regarding their care during pregnancy the way you would are not intuitive enough or informed enough or are somehow doing it wrong. It also can be easy to allow another's comments or opinions stir up doubts and have you call into question your own method of deciding. That's why knowing what works for you is so important. When you're cognizant of the decision-making approach that feels most comfortable to you, then you can feel peaceful and grounded about your choices, regardless of what others think or say.

To follow are stories from women who found their ideal approach.

## Finding your ideal approach

Julia didn't mind getting all kinds of advice from her big family because she knew it was information she could simply store in the back of her mind and use if she needed it. She didn't want to assume she'd need all the suggestions, preferring instead to feel her pregnancy out one step at a time to see what it was like for her and her baby and their circumstances. So she listened to the advice and retained the high-level information so she could go back to the person or recommended resource for details if she needed them. This felt like the best way to take care of herself as she received advice from others.

Along the same lines, Julia decided not to read all the literature available. She didn't want to get into thinking that her pregnancy had to play out a certain way. She wanted to take it one day at a time and tell herself that it is what it is. Julia was conscious of not making any assumptions about what would happen and what information she'd want and need.

Annalise had a different approach. She had specific concerns about the types of information she might hear during her childbirth class. She couldn't imagine *not* going to the class that her doctor recommended because she wanted to get a sense of the care she'd receive in the hospital. Yet, she was anxious about hearing about all the things that could go wrong. Annalise felt that if she listened and absorbed all this information, she'd walk away concerned about potential scenarios that she didn't need to be concerned about. She felt fairly confident and peaceful about her upcoming delivery and didn't want to learn about reasons to be worried.

Annalise talked to her husband about her fears regarding the class. Together, they developed a plan where they would go to the childbirth class together as planned, but when the topic turned to "emergencies" or "interventions," her husband would stay and get the information and Annalise would step out of the room.

Annalise was delighted with this plan because it had begun to feel like a no-win situation. She either had to go to the entire class, complete with information she didn't want to hear, or she was going to have skip the class altogether. To Annalise, the solution she and her husband created allowed for her and for them collectively to have the amount of information that felt ideal for her.

Jennifer, on the other hand, was a researcher. Jumping online and checking statistics, descriptions, suggestions, and user reviews was just what she naturally did for all decisions, whether she was buying herself a pregnancy pillow, dealing with her back pain, or deciding how much caffeine she felt comfortable drinking. She wanted to learn from the experts and learn from others' experiences. Her perspective was that she didn't have to figure it out on her own or make something up. People had already dealt with similar situations or there was data out there allowing her to compare one product to another. Jennifer enjoyed the ease with which she could take this information into account. It seemed so logical to her and gave her the assurance that she had made the best possible choices regarding her own health.

That's not to say she didn't uncover alarming information from time to time. When she was researching how to alleviate her back pain she encountered some disturbing information about women who continued to suffer with back pain years after their pregnancies. She didn't enjoy learning that, yet she knew that without that information, she wouldn't have fully understood her options and associated risks. It was part of the package for her to feel confident with the choices she made. Jennifer's approach was to research until she knew she had a thorough and comparable understanding of the options available. That was what best enabled her to move forward with confidence.

Each of these women used her own methods to determine what would best support her. Whatever works for you is what works for you. You don't have to feel like your plans must be perfectly thought out with a delineated rationale for each of your decisions. You're not going to have to defend them in a court of law. And you don't have to feel like every decision is the result of a perfectly Zen-like experience where you've tapped into the full depths of your maternal intuition. You can do either one, or both, or something in between. You just want to feel good about the care and support you're receiving.

Check in. Which of your approaches to caring for and supporting yourself during pregnancy have felt really good? Why?

## ❀ OKAY, LET'S BE REAL... ❀ ❀ ❀ ❀ ❀ ❀ ❀ ❀ ❀

### I can't think about it anymore!

There may be a moment (or two or more!) when you feel the analyzing and processing has *got* to stop! When you're done checking in with your own thoughts and beliefs and when you're tired of determining what data you want and hunting down that information. You. Have. Had. Enough!

That's just fine. There's value in processing information and having awareness, and there are times when you won't have the energy or drive to do it. Let yourself off the hook for a bit.

Give yourself a break. However long it takes. Allow yourself to be completely removed from serious thinking in that specific area! Even when you're feeling pressure to make a choice or take an action...

## Minimizing stress

Courtney's modus operandi was to be aware of her choices and make sure none of them caused her stress. She understood that stress was not good for a person and especially not for a pregnant person. So, she simply tried to pay attention and notice when she felt herself getting worked up or putting pressure on herself.

One area where she noticed stress creeping in was when she tried to follow advice from pregnancy books to the letter. She believed the distress she felt trying to eat perfectly or eliminate all caffeine, for example, could be more damaging to her than simply giving herself a treat when she craved one. When she noticed that she was starting to get stressed, she told herself to back off and shift tactics.

Workouts were another area where Courtney could feel her stress levels rise. She had been trying to work out at the gym three or four times a week, but it started feeling too structured and strenuous for her. There were times she didn't feel she had the energy to work out, and she was constantly in a dialogue in her own head about whether or not she should go to the gym that day. She didn't like the continual questioning and the pressure she was experiencing. So, she switched gears and focused on simply staying active. She found ways to incorporate activity into her day without creating another "To Do" for herself, like moving around more during her customer service job. She'd walk down the stairs to the Accounts Receivable department on the next floor, rather than using interoffice mail. She'd visit her manager in his office instead of calling or emailing. It was for Courtney a non-pressure way to stay active.

Courtney's simple gut check was to ask herself if she was causing herself stress. If she was, she knew her approaches weren't supportive and nurturing and she needed to find a different way to handle the situation.

We can design our own support team, we can find ways to nourish ourselves, and we can understand how we want to expose ourselves to pregnancy-related information and have that information inform our decisions. These are all great, effective ways to care for ourselves. And, it's important to select care providers who are aligned with what you know best serves you.

## Your beliefs about "official" care providers

There are increasingly more options for the type of care providers you'll use during your pregnancy and childbirth. You can opt to work with a doctor, a midwife, a doula, a birth partner. Maybe you'll also see an acupuncturist or a Reiki Master (who provides energy healing and balancing) or a prenatal massage specialist. There are an infinite number of ways that we can carve out and create our relationships with these types of individuals.

For some, the choice about a primary care provider is super easy. Maybe there's a recommendation from a friend that sounds perfect, or you already have an OB-GYN you love, or you are comfortable knowing that you'll interview the three midwives in your area and choose the one who is the best fit, or you're excited about interviewing doulas with your husband. The details may be different, but the bottom line is that you know you'll make your choice easily.

For others the prospect of making the "right" choice can feel daunting. The number of choices may feel overwhelming. Or you feel the pressure to select the "the best" people to work with during this important and emotional time. Maybe you don't even know where to begin making your choice or what the right criteria should be. The more you explore, the more opportunity you have to get clearer and clearer about what will and what won't work for you.

Often, we are not fully aware of our own assumptions or preconceptions about who the "right" professionals are for us and where those thoughts come from. It's useful to pause and identify the thoughts you have about what's appropriate or acceptable for prenatal care and delivery. For example, you may think that it would be irresponsible and too risky to have a birth outside of a hospital. Or, you may assume that mothers are supposed to deliver babies in the most natural way possible. Maybe you've been led to believe that doctors inside a hospital system are more concerned about liability than what is best for the patient. Maybe you're concerned that others will think you're high maintenance or weird if you hire a doula.

We all have preconceived notions and beliefs like these. And we may not be clear about where they originated. They may have been handed down by our relatives or society or from some experience earlier in your life that you no longer remember. It sometimes takes a good deal of processing to unravel what's present in your mind and heart, and to determine which of those beliefs you want to own and which you want to discard. In doing this, though, you can truly choose for yourself the care providers that are best suited for you.

Early in her pregnancy a friend of a friend suggested to Barb that she meet with her midwife. Barb had never considered working with a midwife. The people she knew went to the OB-GYNs that their general practitioners recommended and that was that. She hadn't questioned that approach; it was simply what people did.

But the suggestion made her reconsider. "Would I want to work with a midwife? Why or why not?" She realized that she had an assumption that only extreme naturalists or people whose faith precluded them from seeking medical intervention went to midwives, although she didn't know where this perspective came from. No one she knew used a midwife and she realized she wasn't clear about the differences between working with a midwife and a doctor or what training and experience midwives had. She got excited about learning more!

In the end, Barb chose to work with a doctor. However, her doctor's practice included both OB-GYNs and midwives so she saw both doctors and midwives throughout her pregnancy and enjoyed doing so. If she hadn't become aware of and explored her assumptions about midwives, she might have felt uncomfortable seeing a midwife in the practice or skipped the experience altogether. She would've missed out on the convenience of seeing whoever was available and the what-proved-to-be-invaluable advice from a midwife who suggested she visit a prenatal chiropractor when her baby was in a breech position. Barb believed her work with this chiropractor shifted the alignment in her body and enabled her baby to turn around.

For each of us, there can be different underlying thoughts or beliefs that impact what we'll consider in terms of care providers. You don't have to be open to a big laundry list of options, certainly, but you don't want to limit yourself, either, especially by influences from outside yourself that unconsciously steer you away from certain choices. So, it's useful to distinguish what you *really* think and feel versus what your assumptions are or how you think others might judge your choices. The way to do that is to give yourself the time and space to explore.

Check in. What do you believe about the care provider options for expectant moms?

How have your beliefs been impacted by what others think or by other external factors?

What care provider options clearly resonate in your core?

## Creating a choice when none exist

It's easy to think that you only have so many options. There are a limited number of doctors or midwives or birthing centers in your area, right? What if none of the options seem aligned with what you want? What happens when the obvious choices don't feel like *your* choices? Is your only option to compromise? Not necessarily.

If there's something telling you that you haven't found your best care provider yet, then keep searching. Look into options you hadn't previously considered. Be open to the unorthodox. Ask questions. Challenge what people are telling you. The more you explore, the more opportunity you have to get clearer and clearer about what does and does not work for you.

When Debra became pregnant about 25 years ago, she knew that she didn't want to experience some of the standard practices at the time like episiotomies and epidurals. She knew from the stories told by her grandmother and mother that natural birth outside a hospital setting was possible. Debra wasn't against delivering in a hospital, she just wanted her delivery to be as natural as possible. She met with a number of OB-GYNs who seemed surprised and somewhat resistant to Debra's desire to forego what were accepted and unquestioned practices at the time.

Debra searched unsuccessfully for the right kind of healthcare provider who was ready and willing to support her choices. Eventually, she found a way to create a situation that worked for her. She met a young resident who was willing to hear her perspectives and wishes and work with her to create the experience she wanted. The resident's supervisor agreed, and the resident and Debra learned together. She shared what she knew to be true from the experiences of the women in her family. He shared what he was learning as a medical resident. Together, they brought past approaches and the latest medical philosophies together in a way that worked for both of them.

Debra was delighted to experience an intact delivery (no episiotomy and no tearing) of her 8 lb. 3 oz. baby in a semi-squat position at the end of her bed. She was proud of herself for trusting that her ideal support partner existed, even when it looked like one didn't. She stayed true to her vision and continued to search until the option revealed itself.

## Do you want to go with the default?

Sometimes your care choices can feel like they are a package deal. Make one decision and you get a lot of default options along with it. For example, you choose your OB-GYN and then it's assumed that you'll deliver at the doctor's usual hospital and that you're on board with the protocols that the hospital typically follows for epidurals or with having residents present because it's a teaching hospital, etc. Or you choose your midwife and then you're expected to deliver at home, naturally in a birthing tub.

It's understandable that certain "defaults" or "assumptions" might go with a care provider choice. For some of us, it might be perfectly fine and even preferable to take some decisions off our plates. It might feel easier when the path is set up, and you can just check in with your own inner guidance to see if it's working for you as it unfolds.

The flip side is that it can feel like you're trapped in all these subsequent choices and you have no option but to go with them. It can feel as if decisions have been made for you.

In those instances, you have the opportunity turn off the autopilot and not go with the "typical" options. You can, for example, have a drug-free delivery in a hospital, you can induce contractions with Pitocin without having an epidural, you can have an epidural under a midwife's care, and you can have a vaginal birth after you've had a c-section. These choices represent those that are often seen as "atypical," and yet they are possible. You can question assumptions and piece together what you most desire.

Or, you may end up choosing everything that is recommended or "standard." That's great too, as long as each choice feels like "your" choice, and that you're choosing consciously or intentionally. You want to be fully aware of why you are going with the default or conversely why you're questioning assumptions.

Let's hear stories from a couple of women who followed their intuition to determine whether the default presented to them would work.

As soon as Dora got pregnant, she intuitively knew that she wanted to give birth in a hospital and that she didn't want to go with her local hospital's standard protocol of administering an epidural. Her friends suggested she deliver at home or at a midwifery center so she could avoid the hospital staff pressuring her to get an epidural. Dora wasn't worried. She knew if she made her wishes clear beforehand then there wouldn't be any confusion. And, she liked the idea of delivering in a hospital and knowing that specialists and pediatricians would be nearby if they were needed. This felt like the best of both worlds to Dora. She was picking and choosing the care options that were the ideal fit for her.

She was proud to be creating and advocating for "her way" because maybe she'd help to make this choice more prevalent. She was jazzed about the idea of potentially exposing hospital personnel to natural birth and expanding their view of what was possible. Dora pieced together the path that felt most in-tune with her desires.

Peg, on the other hand, found she was comfortable with the "default." It seemed as if Peg was the very last of her group of friends to get pregnant. She'd heard plenty of stories about interviewing midwives and doctors and about what the women in her life liked and didn't like about the care practitioners they had. There seemed like a lot to consider and Peg was gearing herself up for an arduous process. She started out by meeting with a midwife that a few of her friends had worked with. Peg immediately felt comfortable with her and knew she didn't have to look any further. Peg felt a little sheepish about not doing more thorough due diligence, but she couldn't imagine not working with this woman. Looking further would have been a waste of time.

Peg presumed that she'd have more deliberation to do later on as she made more choices throughout her pregnancy and in preparation for her delivery. Yet, as she progressed on her journey the choices actually felt easier and easier. As her midwife learned more about her, she was seemingly able to accurately predict what Peg would prefer. Peg just kept going with her midwife's suggestions. It almost seemed too easy. Yet, each time she checked in with herself and questioned whether she felt comfortable with the decisions, the answer was consistently, "Yes." Peg eventually shifted from feeling like she was cheating the system to being extremely appreciative and proud of the synchronistic relationship she had with her midwife.

Check in. Where have you gone with the "default" and how has this worked for you?

Where would you like to question the "default" and why?

The point is that sometimes it feels good to go along with the prescribed path and sometimes it feels better to get more information about the "default" choices. You can choose to question or not question. You can let your feelings be your guide.

## Accepting what's available

What happens when you question the prescribed path and you're told there's not another option? How do you then accept and "feel good" about a choice that is seemingly dictated to you?

Lettie had a very specific need as she sought a doctor's practice. She wanted care providers that felt good to her and that would do a VBAC (vaginal birth after cesarean) after two c-sections. It was difficult, in her area, to find medical or midwifery practices that would do this. It frustrated her to discover that it seemed a facility had to have a VBAC rider on their medical insurance in order to take her as a patient. She felt she was having her choices regarding her care taken away from her.

Although annoyed by this realization, she didn't want to stay in a place of frustration. She chose to accept that she would have another c-section. She'd done it before, so she knew she could do it again. Even though she wouldn't be able to experience the vaginal birth she wanted, she kept her eye on the big picture and reminded herself that she'd still have a healthy and happy baby in the end. And, she could still – inside the parameters of a c-section – create what she wanted, so that's where she focused her attention. She asked herself, "Given this constraint, what do I want to create? What would be most supportive to me?"

Since Lettie was going to be opened up for her c-section and she knew this was her third and last child, she decided to have her tubes tied during the procedure. The response she got from her doctor's office startled her. It was a faith-based practice, and she was told they couldn't conduct that procedure. Lettie was taken aback. She had accepted that she couldn't have the vaginal birth she wanted, she was comfortable with her doctor and the surroundings there, and now she was being told that she couldn't get what she felt was the extra benefit of getting a c-section? This was a non-negotiable for Lettie.

I spoke to Lettie when she was 35 weeks pregnant. She had found a new doctor and there wasn't any angst about it – just this story that she had about her multi-pathed journey to find the doctor that she'd ultimately work with to deliver her baby.

There may be choices that you are locked out of due to hospital practices, particular health risks for you, or other circumstances. When that happens, you can look and ask yourself: "Inside of the boundaries, what do I want to create or choose?"

Check in. What constraints do you know you need to accept so you can move onto creating what you want inside of those constraints?

What do you want to create inside of the constraints?

As we noted in the *Being a Publicly Pregnant Person* chapter, you are not experiencing your pregnancy in a vacuum. When you are choosing your care and support, others are witnessing your choices and are sometimes impacted by them. It can happen: Just when you feel really good about what you're choosing, someone will say something to you, like Sarah did to me. Let's look at how we can deal with the reactions of others.

## When your choice upsets others

Tamara, an RN, decided to work with a midwife in the nearby free-standing midwifery center when she became pregnant. Tamara's belief had always been that unless there's a high risk, pregnancy and childbirth were natural processes. She didn't see a need to seek care at a hospital. Her co-workers were in disbelief. They questioned her, "Why would you go to a midwifery practice when you know the good care that is given here in the hospital?" She grew a little tired of explaining herself, yet felt very comfortable doing so. She was clear in her own mind.

The tough part for Tamara was that her choice made her mom nervous. Conversations with her mom were uncomfortable every time the topic of giving birth came up. She tried asking her mom what would make her feel more comfortable and her mom authentically admitted that nothing short of a delivery in a hospital would reassure her. Tamara explained all the reasons why she felt comfortable with the care and support she'd receive at the center, that she had done her clinicals with a midwifery practice and had been present for many successful births there. She shared story after story, yet her mom remained unconvinced and nervous.

In the end, to stay peaceful and grounded herself, Tamara had to admit that there was nothing further she could do about her mom's anxiety. She repeatedly told herself that it was okay for her to deliver at a midwifery center even though this upset her mom. This was hard.

She and her mom had always been close and had been aligned in nearly all their views up to this point. It felt disappointing and disconcerting that they couldn't talk freely about something that was so important to Tamara. At the same time, Tamara felt reassured by her convictions. She trusted herself and strove to speak about her desires objectively and unapologetically.

The point of Tamara's story is <u>not</u> that you should never allow your decisions about your care to be swayed by others' concerns. It's that others concerns can help you determine your level of conviction. The pushback led Tamara to engage more and more with the inquiry, and she became more and more convinced that delivery at a midwifery center was the choice that best resonated for her. You want to do what best resonates for you, and perhaps others' concerns or fears will alter that. That's okay. In the end, you just want to make sure that it feels like *your* choice.

Check in. What choices are you making that upset others or might upset others?

How do you want to handle their discomfort?

## When your choices are outside the mainstream

Debi made a significant non-mainstream decision when she was pregnant for the second time. During Debi's first birth experience, she discovered that she felt most at peace and cared for when it was just her and her husband in the hospital room. It had been a busy night at the hospital and they were frequently left to themselves. When the staff did come in the room, Debi experienced it as an interruption to her progress and feeling of peace.

Debi was in the whirlpool bathtub in their birthing suite, when a resident came in to check on her. The resident felt the baby's head crowning and appeared to panic. Suddenly, the room filled with medical staff. They got Debi out of the bathtub, onto the bed and told her not to push because the doctor had not yet arrived. Much of what occurred in this phase of her delivery didn't quite make sense to Debi.

When Debi was pregnant again five years later, she knew she wanted a different birth experience. She wanted the second birth to be more about her family and about the sacredness that she and her husband had felt when they were alone in the hospital the first time.

Her first step was to contact the two midwives in her area. One, with whom she felt a great connection, was unfortunately not available when Debi was due. The second did not feel like a good fit in Debi's view. Despite not finding a local midwife, Debi was still not ready to compromise.

She then explored something many of us might not even consider; she began to research having her baby at home unassisted except for her husband. A do-it-yourself birth, if you will. As Debi investigated, she became more and more convinced that they could do this and that it felt right. After all, women were having babies long before hospitals were around!

She knew that not everyone would share in her excitement. She explained, "We understood that a lot of people would be freaked out by our choice to not work with a care provider, so we tried to keep it on the down low." However, this proved to be quite challenging since one of the most common questions a pregnant women gets is, "Where are you delivering?" One woman who homeschooled her children went so far as to advise Debi not to tell *anyone* what she was planning. Getting this advice from someone who was undertaking a non-mainstream endeavor impacted Debi. It was a sign of how much fear there is about things that are not commonplace.

Debi understood the fear and knew that at one point, she might have been skeptical, too. Yet, her experience with her first pregnancy and her research gave her a level of comfort with the idea. As others' expressed their unease, Debi knew it could be easy to get engulfed in their fear so she kept silently asking herself, "Are you afraid? Have you heard something that makes you want to change your mind?" As her answers kept coming back, "No, this still feels right," she felt increasingly comfortable and secure with their path.

Debi's silent questions to herself can remind all of us that we are the ones that need to feel confident and secure about our care and support. No one else. We can take others' feelings into consideration, certainly. And, those considerations might alter what feels best to us. Yet, in the end, we want our care and support choices to clearly resonate as the best choices for us.

In the stories shared in this chapter, each woman explored her own belief systems, trusted her own knowledge and feelings, learned from her experiences, and did her best job – with the information and self-awareness that she had – to make the choices about her care and support that worked best for her.

## ❋ Choosing Your Care and Support ❋ ❋ ❋ ❋ ❋

You get to choose the care and support you receive during your pregnancy. It's up to you to create what you want. Others can't read your mind. And, remember, the act of asking for support is not a weak one. It's a sign of strength and confidence and demonstrates you're gracious enough to let others contribute.

* You don't have to know it all or do it all. You can create your unique support team.

* Look beyond the support that's going to "get you by" to what will truly nourish you.

* Know the type and level of information that you want to feel comfortable making a choice.

* Pay attention to your approach and mindset and ensure they are supportive for you.

* You can intentionally choose the "defaults" or "assumptions" that go with a choice you've made or you can choose to question them.

* At times there are constraints around what you can choose. When this is the case, do what you can to accept this choice and create what you want inside of the choice.

* Recognize that others may not know what you know. They may not understand why some of your choices work for you.

Check In. What is most important for you to remember as you choose your care and support?

# Loving How You Look

It's quite fashionable these days to be pregnant! There are designer label maternity clothes. There are clever t-shirts to publicize your pregnant status. Pop culture magazines are forever on a celebrity baby bump watch! Actresses, singers, and models are not going into hiding during the nine months of pregnancy; they are out and about flaunting their maternity fashions and growing bellies. Expectant moms at workplaces everywhere are assembling professional, well-fitting, classy wardrobes. We're living in a time when it can be fashionable to be pregnant and where it can be chic to show off a pregnant shape.

In the *Being a Publicly Pregnant Person* chapter, I asked how you wanted to *be* as a pregnant person and we explored the adjectives you'd use to describe the best version of the pregnant you. In this chapter, the core questions are: How do you want to *look*? What are the adjectives you'd use to describe your *image*? How can you embrace the way you look and the way you feel about how you look? Your responses to these questions might stem directly from how you want to *be* as a pregnant person. Yet, what you process when you consider the inquiries in this chapter might be quite different.

As expectant moms we have the opportunity to feel just as fashionable, professional, sexy, hot, punk-ish, athletic, and/or well-put-together as any other time in our lives. However, pregnancy can be a time when we feel like we lose a little bit (or a lot) of ourselves and possibly our va-va-voom. Many pregnant women feel like it's no longer appropriate or possible to feel sexy or hot while pregnant. We might think that we don't even look like ourselves; like our entire image has changed.

It can seem like there are only certain images that are possible for pregnant women, images like matronly, cute, girl next door, responsible, and wholesome. Picture the docile, angelic woman in the rocking chair wearing muted pastel tones with her hand on her belly. And, if this isn't your image, what are you to do? What if your image is punk, bold, bright, hot, or sexy? What if it is powerful, professional, and in charge? How do you evolve your pregnancy image into one that is aligned with who you truly are? These are the questions presented in this chapter.

I remember thinking that the best I could hope for while pregnant was "cute." That pulling off "beautiful" or "hot" – which I had heard from my husband in my pre-pregnant days – would just be impossible. I believed I couldn't simultaneously have a swollen pregnant belly and be considered "hot"…not by anyone's standards.

Three months into my pregnancy we got invited to a wedding where a lot of our friends from college, whom we hadn't seen in years, would attend. I got to thinking, "I want to look *good* at that wedding." When I figured out I was going to be nine months pregnant for the event, my immediate reaction was, "Yikes! I am going to be huge! How am I possibly going to look good?"

This late-in-my-pregnancy wedding proved to be a valuable incentive for me. I felt vain admitting – to even myself – that I was on a campaign to look good because I was seeing people I hadn't seen since college. Yet, that was the truth and it became a healthy motivator to stay fit. And, I began to realize that although my commitment stemmed from a seemingly superficial desire, it launched a number of extremely useful activities and inquiries for me. It confirmed for me early on my desire to determine the best styles and fabrics for my pregnant body. It got me involved in understanding my evolving shape and image. I actively owned up to the fact that I cared about how I looked, and I did what I could to feel good about how I looked.

Expectant moms have continued to confirm for me that it's okay – and can even be transformational – to want to look beautiful and sexy during pregnancy. It doesn't have to be all babies and booties and nursery decorating. It doesn't have to be mom fully sacrificing her body and how she sees and knows herself. There can be both. We can do what we need to do for our unborn babies *and* portray the image we want while we're doing so. In fact, I think it's part of the ever-evolving lesson of how not to lose ourselves inside of the role of being a parent. We have the opportunity to be ourselves as a parent. This can start (or continue) with discovering the pregnancy image you want to create.

## Discovering your pregnancy image

Anita had always been an athlete. She was known in all her circles as a fit, athletic person. Even people she'd meet for the first time would comment that she looked like she was in great shape or really strong. She'd get an occasional, "Wow, I think you could take my husband!"

Anita enjoyed this persona. When she became pregnant she worried that she'd lose this part of who she was. She didn't think she'd be viewed in the same way. It distressed to her to think that she'd lose a part of her identity for a number of months.

When Anita became fully cognizant of these concerns, she considered what she wanted to do about them and came up with a couple of options. She could prepare herself for the idea that she wouldn't be viewed as athletic for a period of time. She could look forward to fully reinstating her athletic image post-pregnancy. She could make a point of talking more about the sports and physical activities she was involved in so people would continue to realize that she was an active athlete.

Yet, what Anita realized she needed to do more than anything else was to change her own view that a pregnant body couldn't be an *athletic* body. She was an athlete, right? She'd continue to be one during her pregnancy. Her body, by definition, was going to be an athletic one throughout her pregnancy. She started to look forward to observing the changes in her body. Her "everyday" body looked different than others. Her pregnant body would, too. She got excited about creating a new pregnancy image, and was able to achieve what was most desirable to her: a muscular, fit, pregnant body that people continued to notice.

Colette was looking forward to gaining a new image during her pregnancy. She had been overweight for a number of years and being pregnant meant having what she called a "legitimate reason" to have a big belly. She would now be *pregnant,* not *fat.* She looked forward to shaking her previous body image issues and living in a body that was supposed to be big in the breasts and belly. She was hopeful that pregnancy would provide a shift in thinking that would feel better to her.

At the same time, some anxiety snuck in about getting even bigger in places where she didn't want to gain weight. If that happened, instead of feeling purposeful and curvy in all the right places, she was concerned she'd feel pregnant *and* fat. As she acknowledged this fear, she intuitively knew it was time for a whole new mindset.

She started to spend time looking for and appreciating aspects of her pregnancy shape that she enjoyed. She noticed, for example, and for perhaps the first time, that her hips were in perfect proportion to her shoulders and body size. She also talked with women about how their bodies looked and felt after pregnancy. And, although not everyone she spoke with had seemingly positive results to report, Colette held onto the idea that her post-pregnancy body was likely to be different than her pre-pregnancy body. She looked forward to witnessing the differences and having an influence on the changes and how she viewed them.

Colette emerged from pregnancy appreciative of the changes her curvy body had made and knowing that her body could continue to shift and look differently. She wasn't locked into her pre-pregnancy "fat" body image. She had hope that she could continue to positively shift her self-image.

Check in. How do you want to look? What is your desired pregnancy image?

How do you want to feel about how you look?

None of us can know how our bodies will change and look during our pregnancies. In fact, during a second pregnancy, our bodies might react completely differently than they did previously. This can be daunting – not knowing what's coming. It can be useful to proactively consider how we're going to deal with our constantly changing and somewhat unpredictable bodies. What mindsets do you think will work for you? What approaches?

## Focus on physical aspects that work for you…

When Andrea was beginning to think about getting pregnant the first time, she dreaded the changes her body would go through. She hated the idea of her body changing in ways she couldn't predict and of feeling out of control. And, she too, was concerned about fitting into what she called a "traditional" pregnancy image. She didn't consider herself matronly. She didn't want to look matronly. She didn't want to be that wholesome, boring-looking person on the cover of some pregnancy books.

Andrea was clear about what she didn't want. Then, she started to ask herself: "How *do* I want to look?" She wasn't sure. She couldn't get past the stereotypical images she had of pregnant women. Instead she had to back up and start with the question: What, physically, do I like about the idea of being pregnant?

Andrea realized that she loves trying new things and loves it when she and others stretch traditional boundaries to do something in a unique way. The physical aspect of pregnancy that she could get jazzed about was the idea that she could grow a person inside of her. She could carry another person around with her for nine months! It was fascinating to Andrea. It led her to a place of, "Look at me! Isn't this cool?" From here she could set aside her concerns and consider how she wanted to look and dress as she was accomplishing this miraculous task. She wanted to dress in much the same way as she had prior to being pregnant. And, she didn't want to shy away from form-fitting clothing that would accentuate her baby bump. Her awe and enthusiasm about what a woman's body was capable of started to naturally show through. She was able to create the image she wanted to portray.

As LuAnn moved into her second trimester, her body changed quickly and she suddenly felt sloppy and fat. This was primarily due to the size of her breasts. They grew more than a cup size and her clothes, as a result, hung "way out there, seemingly making her appear big everywhere. LuAnn had never been a thin girl. She'd always been more curvy and voluptuous, but this was just too much in LuAnn's eyes. How was she going to feel good about herself and how she looked when she looked like this?! For a while, LuAnn felt really insecure about her appearance. Then two things happened. One, LuAnn got to thinking, "What if I have a daughter inside my belly? What am I teaching her if I am judging my self-worth based on how I look?" And, two, she had a friend tell her she was so lucky because her ankles weren't swelling at all. This inspired a new approach for LuAnn. She had been so busy lamenting about how her boobs and torso looked that she completely overlooked how great her legs looked. Her new wardrobe plan was to accentuate her legs!

The next day, LuAnn went shopping and purchased more skirts and dresses with interesting hemlines that would bring attention to her legs. And, she used this as an excuse to buy some rockin' new shoes. And, it worked! Throughout the rest of her pregnancy she got compliments about her great shoes and her skinny ankles. She heard, "I can't believe you're wearing those high heels! You're amazing. You look amazing!"

LuAnn loved the idea that she had found a way to focus on what was working for her physically, rather than obsessing about what she didn't enjoy. She believed she was already setting a good example for her daughter (she did have a girl!). She demonstrated how to not obsess about a self-proclaimed body flaw, and to, instead, acknowledge and leverage positives and strengths.

Check in. What physical aspects of pregnancy do you personally like?

How can you focus on or accentuate what's working?

## Pregnancy glow

When we're pregnant, our hormone levels are shifting and creating changes. The affects on our physical appearance vary. Some women get that glow about them. For other women, their skin may become drier, oilier, rosier, softer, and/or break out in blemishes. How will you prepare for or react to any changes you may experience?

When Natalie was expecting, she was simply bursting with pride and giddiness. She had been trying to get pregnant for a while and couldn't have been more delighted to watch her growing belly, to shop for maternity clothes, and to be noticeably and obviously pregnant. Her friends and family could easily see this. It was written all over her face. Natalie was told repeatedly, "You are just glowing!" This was exceptionally fun for some time, and then she noticed a shift. After a while people almost seemed to get fed up with Natalie. She heard, "You're not supposed to look this happy when you're pregnant!" "It's not right. You should be getting acne, not glowing like a little kid."

The comments were upsetting and a little confusing to Natalie. Why couldn't others just be happy about how she felt and looked? Why did they act like this was the "wrong" or "abnormal" way to look?

Natalie decided there was nothing she could do about her healthy-looking skin and she also wasn't going to tone down her enthusiasm that seemingly caused her to radiate happiness. She told herself that she shouldn't have to apologize for being happy and looking good. She was ecstatic and was going to act like it. After declaring this for herself, Natalie found others' negative comments and reactions to be more amusing than annoying. In some cases, she felt real compassion for the other person. She realized that the comments probably represented more of a longing or disappointment within the other person, rather than saying anything about Natalie.

Erin, on the other hand, had terrible skin during her pregnancy. She had not been expecting to have oily skin and breakouts, and she was disappointed and frustrated when it showed up. Each morning she'd look in the mirror and think "yuck."

Erin had to find a way to stop obsessing about her acne. Usually, she wasn't a big makeup gal. For years she'd been someone who could waltz out of the house with barely any makeup on and look great. She finally stopped lamenting about her skin and said, "Okay, this is the time for me to learn how to apply makeup!" She went to makeup counters, got tips from professionals and friends, and learned how to cover up blemishes and accentuate her eyes without looking too "made up" or "cakey." She actually started having fun playing with colors and her application brushes. She got into something she never thought she would be interested in.

During her first pregnancy, Melissa's complexion stayed the same; yet, she noticed her hair got fuller and shinier. She thought it was due to the prenatal vitamins she was taking. Regardless of the reason, she was going to enjoy it. She continued to grow her hair longer and longer, going to the salon frequently to freshen up the style. In her second trimester, she added blonder highlights. She found herself spending more time on her primping in the morning and enjoyed feeling pretty with noticeably awesome hair! She jumped in with enthusiasm and made the most of an unexpected change.

Check In. What mindsets and approaches will work for you as your physical appearance changes in ways you may or may not expect?

## Stop comparing!

Samantha confessed that it was hard for her to accept the weight she gained during pregnancy. Before she got pregnant, she thought that pregnancy weight gain wasn't a big deal. You simply dealt with it for a limited period of time and sucked it up for the sake of your baby. But as someone who bloated easily and quickly during pregnancy, she started to realize that it was one thing to watch others gain weight and quite another to experience it yourself. As soon as she was pregnant, she began gaining weight fast and retaining water. By her second month, she couldn't fit into any of her "regular" clothes. It bothered her deeply to get so big so quickly. She felt enormous, out of control. and worried about just how big she was going to get!

The books she read told her she should expect, in the first trimester, to gain a lot less weight than she had. She was comparing herself to others and to statistics and not enjoying how she felt about herself. At times, she felt almost panicked at what might be coming.

Finally, it occurred to her that she needed to stop. She told herself to stop reading, stop Googling, stop comparing. She reminded herself that of course she was going to gain weight. She needed to gain weight because she was pregnant. It was all for a good cause.

Samantha knew she had to concentrate her thoughts on something else. She started focusing on the time when she'd first feel her baby moving inside her. She knew once she could connect with her baby in that more tangible way, it'd be easier for her to appreciate what she was doing as an expectant mom, instead of obsessing about weight gain.

Shifting her thoughts helped alleviate some of her angst and frustration. Her dislike of her weight gain never fully went away. Yet, she did learn to keep her comparative, competitive mind in check by tuning into her baby and her baby's health and movement. This helped her to feel better about her pregnancy and herself.

Check In. How will you keep yourself from engaging in unhealthy comparisons?

## OKAY, LET'S BE REAL...

But I want to compare, if I'm gonna come out on top!

We don't want to engage in unhealthy comparisons that will leave us feeling bad and "less than."

Yet...let's get real. There are times when you're going to need a good esteem boost. If you just read that some celebrity gained twice as much weight as you, make the comparison and be proud! If something is going better for you than it does for most pregnant women, do a victory dance in your living room. Give yourself as many props as you can in the privacy of your own home or head. Make the comparisons in your mind that make you look good!

If you're going to come out on top – and you're not outwardly putting anyone else down – go ahead and compare away! Give yourself some moments to feel "better than." Feel great about what you're achieving. Own it and celebrate it!

# Working the maternity clothes

In order to show up looking good and feeling good at that wedding I mentioned earlier, I had to do some exploration with maternity clothes. The body parts I accentuated on my non-pregnant body were not the same ones I wanted to accentuate while I was expecting. I no longer had a trim waistline. Yet, I did have some new – previously nonexistent – cleavage to show off. I had to retrain myself because the kinds of clothes that I had gravitated towards for decades no longer worked for me. It was well worth spending some time and effort to better understand the best styles and shapes for my pregnant body.

Adriana subscribed to *People* magazine and always enjoyed looking at how celebrities dressed during their pregnancies. She found it fascinating to see who would drape themselves in lots of fabric, who would show their bare-skinned bellies, and who would wear form-fitted clothes. Adriana decided that she preferred snug clothing that showed off the pregnant belly shape. She felt that adding more fabric made people look bigger than they were. When she became pregnant, she knew she'd want to wear tailored looks.

To her surprise, it took her a little while to get used to the feel of the tailored looks she liked so much. Her desire at times was to camouflage, not wear the tight clothing that showed everything! So, she reminded herself of her opinions and checked in with herself asking, "Are these still my preferences? Does the snug clothing actually work for me?" She decided that, yes, she did prefer the tailored look on others and on herself. It was just something she needed to get used to. So, she took her time choosing clothes. And she would wear the snuggest clothing out with her good friends first and get their seal of approval before she took them more public. In the end, Adriana felt great about how she stepped into a new comfort zone with her clothing.

Check in. How will you get to know your pregnancy shape?

What will you do to determine how to best show your style during pregnancy?

## Working with the clothes you've got

Amanda didn't like the idea of maternity clothes. Her weight had fluctuated a few times throughout her life and she already had – she thought – too many clothes hanging in her closet that didn't fit. She didn't want to buy another set of clothes during her pregnancy that would eventually fall into that same category. At the same time, she wanted to look well-put-together and professional during her pregnancy.

Her pregnancy shape wasn't all that different from her everyday shape. As she reached different stages of her pregnancy, she took time on the weekends to try on clothes and make sure she had enough workable outfits for the week. She found that some previously "too big" shirts now worked nicely as "maternity" tops. She plowed through her closet and found she could use many of her current items.

In the later stages of her pregnancy, Amanda did need to break down and buy more skirts and pants than she had originally imagined. Even then, she leveraged her existing wardrobe by making sure her purchases coordinated with tops she already owned. She was proud of how she had stretched (literally and figuratively!) the clothes she had to minimize her spending on maternity wear.

I understand Amanda's perspective. We're not with bigger bellies for all that long – a few months. It doesn't seem feasible or practical to many to purchase a complete wardrobe for that amount of time. *And*, just because we're pregnant, doesn't mean we don't want to feel well-put-together and sophisticated, sexy, sweet, sassy, or whatever "s" you're going for. This is not a time for scraping by with items that don't feel good. That's not an "s" you should desire! On the other hand, many would argue it's also not a time for unnecessary spending. There's a newborn baby on the way and this is going to impact the household budget. How do you strike the balance between feeling confident and comfortable about the clothes you wear out and feeling good about the dollars you've spent on maternity clothes?

## Striking a balance

How much you spend on your maternity wardrobe and what you spend it on is obviously a personal choice. Some women really love shopping – any kind of shopping. Some expectant moms decide that pregnancy is a time to splurge. They consider it a time when it's really important to feel confident and comfortable, and they give themselves permission to spend some dollars to help in this endeavor. Other women feel guilty about buying items over a certain dollar amount. Some expectant moms may feel bad spending any money on themselves, especially when it's for a clothing item that'll only be worn for a few months.

It's good to know yourself. Are you someone who tends to overspend and then feel badly about it? Are you someone who always resists splurging on yourself, even when you can afford to? Acknowledge your typical tendencies and consider if and how you'd like to shift them during pregnancy. Giving your spending habits and perspectives intentional consideration can help you determine your ideal balance for spending what you want and being able to wear what you want.

Check in. Do you tend to reside on the over-spending or the under-spending side of the continuum?

How will you strike a balance between having a great wardrobe during pregnancy and not spending more money than desirable?

## Discovering *your* approach to maternity clothes

What is going to be your approach to maternity clothes? Will you buy a few high-quality staples? Will you look to acquire items very similar to what you have now? Are you open to acquiring and/or purchasing used items? Will you think about each trimester differently? There are many different methods that can work.

Prepare yourself that your approach to your maternity wardrobe is likely to be different than the one you have for your everyday wardrobe because you're probably not going to purchase or acquire another whole closet full of clothes. And, even if you did, your body size and shape will be changing throughout your pregnancy. So, it's a dynamic process!

During our pregnancies, no one expects us to be Kate Middleton, wearing a new ensemble every time we are seen in public! I think it's fair to say that we can repeat clothing items much more frequently while we're expecting. Meghan had a favorite skirt that looked so good and was so comfortable that she admitted to wearing it all the time throughout her third trimester. Winona had a black top that she loved and she'd just switch up the accessories she wore with it each time, creating different looks with her necklaces, scarves, and earrings. Amy literally made a note about what she wore to work every day, so she could ensure she was varying her limited ensembles as much as she possibly could.

Molly was completely delighted and surprised one day when she showed up at a client site and one of the women waltzed up and handed her a shopping bag. "These are for you," the client said. Molly looked in the bag and saw a maternity shirt and a maternity sweater. The woman explained that she felt two items could make a huge difference in a pregnant woman's wardrobe. So she was giving away two items to every pregnant woman she knew. She didn't want the items back. She just wanted Molly to make good use of them. The woman added, "If they don't work for you, please just pass them along to someone who can use them."

Molly did get a lot of wear out of her client's gift and wholeheartedly agreed with her client: two items could go a long way! So, Molly subsequently did two things. She started asking her friends, who had been pregnant recently, if they had just a couple of items they wouldn't mind loaning her. Her friends responded generously! Molly filled out most of her casual wardrobe with loaners from friends. She was so glad she'd asked. Then, after her second and final pregnancy, Molly began parceling out her maternity wardrobe. It felt great to support a number of other women in having more varied maternity attire.

Most weekends Jessica would try on her outfits for the week, making sure she had five outfits that fit her well, felt comfortable, and looked good. She didn't want to have a morning where she'd get out of the shower, put something on and hate how it looked or felt. She knew this would plunge her into a bad mood as she frantically tried to find something that fit or looked better. If she reviewed her clothes on the weekend, then she'd know she was set and she could look forward to getting dressed each morning. This is a smart practice. Our bodies change frequently during pregnancy and what worked two weeks ago might no longer work. Re-assessing our wardrobes throughout our pregnancies could be useful and help us avoid any last minute panics about having nothing to wear!

Jen got great brand name clothes at affordable prices by shopping on eBay. She found women selling brand-new items and gently used clothes! By searching for the exact brands and styles she'd seen in top-end stores, she got a handful of professional clothes online that were distinctive and made her feel great, without spending a fortune.

Liza's approach was to shop for pants at high-end boutiques. It was important to her to have pants that fit over her hips comfortably, were made of a high-quality fabric, and had the adjustable waistline that she could slowly let out in her third trimester. She invested in and got a ton of wear out of the expensive black, brown, and grey striped pants she bought. Liza paired them with tops from moderate-priced or discount stores. She felt this was the best way to get the most of her money and have a wardrobe that was appropriate for a range of casual to formal events.

Anita loved the clothes they had at the maternity shop in her town. She started out by going in and buying all the blouses and skirts that she loved best. She soon realized that she needed to be a little more thoughtful. By purchasing items in unique colors and patterns, she couldn't wear them frequently enough. They were too memorable! Anita decided to get more strategic and added some classic styles in solid colors to her wardrobe, so she could mix and match her pieces in a larger variety of ways.

For Melissa, it felt good to wait as long as possible to move into maternity clothes. It was a point of pride for her. For some reason – and she admitted it was probably an egotistical one – she wanted to be able to say that she hadn't started wearing maternity clothes until month four or even month five. It became a sort of game for her. Did she still have clothes that fit or that she could make work with a rubber band stretched from button to button hole to expand the waistline? Could she simply buy a larger size? She didn't feel that the majority of maternity clothes matched her style, so she wore normal clothes as long as she could.

And, she was cognizant of the idea that perhaps she was foolishly and pridefully avoiding maternity clothes for irrational reasons. She kept checking in with herself: "Am I being silly? Or is this game really working for me (for whatever reason)? Would it be easier to give in and move into maternity clothes?" Melissa felt she was being self-aware and kept herself in regular clothes until the beginning of her sixth month. Then, she found some great styles that accentuated her growing belly in ways that worked for her. In the end she was proud she played the game she wanted to play for as long as it worked for her.

Check in. How will you approach the needed change in clothing?

What approaches and mindsets feel good to you?

## More than the clothes, it's the attitude

Regardless of the clothes you put on, how you think about your pregnant body will heavily influence how you feel about how you look. Your attitude is as important – if not more so – than your actual maternity wardrobe in enabling you to love how you look.

Georgia was proud of her pregnant belly and wore clothes such that her bare belly would show. She was usually a midriff-baring lady and she saw no reason to change. She had a relaxed, free-flowing style and being comfortable was important to her. She often wore short tops and billowing skirts, and she wanted to continue to do so during her pregnancy. Georgia caught some seemingly scornful looks thrown her way, and her neighbor would ask her if she was going to change before they left for lunch. Yet, this was her style and she wanted it to continue to be. Others weren't going to make her cover up!

When Georgia traveled to Mexico during her pregnancy, she perceived a much different reaction to her exposed belly. Women's faces would light up as they looked her up and down. People exclaimed that she was beautiful and complimented her clothing. She felt others' approval and was treated like a Queen. She marveled at and enjoyed the reverence that the Mexican culture had for her role as expectant mother. This experience confirmed her desire to embrace – and often expose – her growing belly.

Gretchen was the most comfortable in a bikini when she was pregnant. Her two pregnancies were the only times when she wasn't walking along sucking in her stomach. She vividly remembered one stroll down the beach on vacation with her husband and daughter when she was eight months pregnant with her son. She felt so proud of her growing family. She'd been taking good care of herself during the pregnancy. Her body wasn't perfect by any stretch. Yet, she was so happy to have her belly sticking out there. Two women came up to her on that walk to compliment her. One said that her shape was so cute and the other said she was glad to see her in a bikini. Gretchen was simply glowing. It was a type of rock star experience for Gretchen and she loved the attention she was getting. And, she was glad that she allowed herself to revel in that attention.

Laura had a tendency to put on weight easily. She anticipated that she was going to be a little round balloon, and she was ready for that. She would tell herself, "Okay, the weight I will gain will be the weight I will gain. I'm going to let it be." She was gearing herself up with an accommodating attitude.

However, it never happened. She didn't balloon up. In her pregnancy, she became slim and elegant. All her hormones decided to work in a beautiful orchestrated manner. Her skin was great, her body thinned out, and she felt perfectly proportioned when she had expected the exact opposite.

People started profusely complimenting her, saying "Wow Laura, you look fantastic! You look better than ever." These comments caused Laura to pause and think, "What? I looked awful before?" She was viewing these as back-handed compliments. Then she caught herself. She had been preparing herself to look like a little round balloon, and when that didn't happen, she started worrying over someone complimenting her trim body! She recognized she was trading one concern for another and decided to shift back to her original mindset and let it be. In fact, she embraced people's reactions and soaked in the compliments. She appreciated this pregnant body she never thought she'd have and viewed it as such a gift.

Chris experienced something entirely different. She was normally trim with a good natural metabolism. She hadn't been expecting the all-over weight gain she experienced. She was annoyed and disgusted. This wasn't the image she was used to projecting – someone who couldn't control her weight and body shape. She felt like everyone was watching her body grow and was seeing her fail. She felt like she was failing, and very publicly. Chris didn't like it and it was impacting how she felt about herself. Getting dressed each morning became an exercise in self-loathing. She knew she needed to snap out of the mindset she was in.

Chris asked herself: "How can I project *my* usually confident and bold image?" It was hard to answer this question, because she felt anything but confident and bold. Yet, she knew it started with continuing to wear bold colors. That didn't necessarily mean wearing hot pink from neck to knee, but she could pair dark clothing with a splash of her usual colors in all the outfits she wore. And, she decided she'd be one of those gals who ballooned up during pregnancy and then moved right back into shape. This mindset helped her accept her weight gain and pregnant shape. It gave her a way to deal with her pregnant body without disliking it and gave her something to look forward to post-pregnancy. This was what kept her in the best spirits.

Check In. What attitude about your pregnancy body and wardrobe will best serve you?

## Utilitarian versus sexy

For many women, the utility of the pregnant body – the idea that the body's purpose is to house and nourish a fetus – can detract from a feeling of sexiness. When you're pregnant, your body is changing in hundreds of ways to enable the development of a baby. These changes are for the baby. They aren't necessarily for you and your sexual prowess. It's easy to begin to feel like a baby factory, rather than like a sexy, sensual being.

However, it is possible to make a baby and make your partner hot for you at the same time! Tina was someone who always really enjoyed her sexual side and her sex life with her husband. When her body started changing during pregnancy, she began to feel less desirable. Her boobs were bigger than she wanted and she didn't think the new curves on her belly and hips were very attractive. She was feeling flabby and floppy and decidedly not like her normal sensual self. She resigned herself to the idea that her body was not her own for a while and that she had to step back from what she wanted in order to allow her body to do what it needed to do. Yet, as she was telling herself this, it didn't feel good, it didn't ring true. She'd found ways to maintain a strong, healthy body image at other times in her life, why couldn't she now? She shifted her thinking into this inquiry: "How can I be a baby-making machine *and* feel sexually desirable?" Tina began to answer this one body part at a time.

First, she got herself a couple of racy bras that would hold the girls in place during bedroom playtime. It was different. She was used to nakedness being the most desirable. Yet, she got into seeing herself literally and enticingly pouring out of the bras she'd bought.

Her husband was excited to see what she'd purchased. Things were changing in ways she hadn't expected or originally wanted, but they were interesting changes. She began to understand that these shifts were good for their overall sex life and relationship. Both of their bodies were going to change in shape over time. And when this happened or they incurred new physical restrictions, she didn't want to stop exploring how they could keep their chemistry strong.

Tina also experimented with body lotions and oils to promote skin firmness and reduce the chance of stretch marks. She's not sure how much these worked, yet she enjoyed paying attention to her body and playing with different scents. She was getting acquainted with her body and her sexiness in a whole new way. This helped Tina during her pregnancy, certainly, and she was actually most excited about what her new-found insights meant for her future. She knew it would serve her and her husband throughout the rest of their lives to know that they could continue – regardless of circumstances – to find new and creative ways to embrace their bodies and turn each other on.

Mindy felt like an alien had taken over her body during her pregnancy. Physically, it felt odd and disconcerting to her. As her pregnancy progressed, she felt resentful that her body was seemingly no longer her own. She loved the baby inside of her, yet she didn't love what was happening to her body. It wasn't that she specifically disliked certain aspects of her pregnant body. She enjoyed how her boobs were fuller. Her belly was growing at a nice pace. She had a few blemishes on her skin, but nothing that wasn't easily disguised with makeup. People told her that she was lucky, that she had a cute pregnant body. She couldn't disagree. It just didn't feel like *her* body. It bothered her that she didn't seem to have a say in what was going on. Her body was doing what it was doing, acting in new and different ways, and she was powerless – she believed – to stop it or alter it.

Mindy recognized her irritation early on and found a couple friends with whom she could talk freely about her body takeover frustrations. This allowed her to acknowledge what she did like about her pregnant body and helped her get clear that it was the "out of control" aspect of the changes she was experiencing that annoyed her most. She focused on what she could control: her hair, the design of her clothes, the way she held and carried herself, and so on. This helped her feel like she was evolving in tandem with her body, rather than being a victim of a takeover.

Check in. Do you believe your body can be highly utilitarian and super sexy at the same time? Why or why not?

What would you like to believe?

## ✿ OKAY, LET'S BE REAL… ✿ ✿ ✿ ✿ ✿ ✿ ✿ ✿ ✿

What makes you think you can touch my body?

What is it about the pregnant belly that makes people – even complete strangers – think they can touch it?! We'd never dream of walking up to a non-pregnant person and putting our hands on her abdomen. Why do some people think it is okay simply because there's a baby in there? If we are sharing our bellies with a baby, then we're automatically sharing it with everyone? I don't think so!

Let's get real and spread the word: The belly is still one of a woman's body parts, and you need permission to touch it.

## Working out your workouts

Physical fitness can be an important factor in helping you to feel good. You carry yourself more confidently when you know you're being physically active in a way that works for you. Pregnancy is a time when you may need to reassess what level and types of activity are most appropriate and what mindsets will best serve you. How can you make sure you don't overdo or under-do in the area of physical activity? How can you discover the level of activity that works best for you physically and mentally and leaves you feeling good?

Fitness mindsets for expectant moms can vary greatly. You want to be gentle and wholly honest with yourself and discover the perspective that's going to empower you. If you're not one who has exercised in the past, it's not realistic to expect yourself to do regular prenatal yoga and gym visits when you become pregnant. On the other hand, maybe pregnancy provides the perfect motivator to begin an activity you've only contemplated previously. Maybe you'll need to slow down your fitness regime. Or, maybe you're empowered by the idea of sustaining what you've always done as you move into your pregnancy.

Talk to your care providers, and first and foremost, listen to yourself and your body. If you pay close attention, you can know if you're putting unnecessary pressure on yourself, if your body wants you to increase your movement, or if you can't maintain a program you started. Tune into your body sensations and, at the same time, your thoughts and feelings. These can be your guides to the workouts that work best for you!

## One size does not fit all

Nancy knew that there was not a one-size-fits-all fitness regime that would be perfect for all pregnant women. She knew she'd have to determine for herself what was appropriate for her. She said, "It's actually liberating. There's no model." She kept telling herself that all she could do was choose a path and if it didn't work out, that would be okay. She'd then just have to try something different.

Two months after the birth of her first child, Nancy started going to personal training classes. The classes got her right back into shape and she felt great.

When Nancy found out she was pregnant again, she told her personal trainer right away. At that point, she believed it would feel best to keep working out with her trainer who had prenatal fitness experience and information. Her trainer had safely and comfortably ramped up her post-partum workouts, so Nancy wanted her support on the other side. She trusted her trainer and she trusted herself to listen to her body.

At about six months, Nancy geared herself up for the idea that she'd need to start modifying certain exercises and movements. She wanted to continue to do as much as she could without quitting completely, unless she had to. She knew it would be a big disappointment physically and emotionally to no longer work with her trainer if she had to stop. She'd sorely miss the connection with her body and she'd miss the close relationship with her trainer. However, Nancy was committed to listening to her body and doing what worked. She continued to remind herself that all she could do was choose a path and stay on it as long as it continued to make sense, and to switch paths when her body needed a change.

Nancy was intentional about keeping her eye on the bigger picture – a healthy baby – and telling herself it was okay to change her approach at any time, and enjoying what she could along the way.

## Creating a pregnancy fitness regime

Shortly after moving to London to establish herself as a successful personal trainer, Nisha found out she was pregnant. This was unexpected. At first, Nisha wasn't even willing to look at how this might impact her business goals. She continued to focus on building her business brand and finding clients. She soon found herself working 15 hours a day, not eating properly, not yet making enough money, and under a heck of a lot of stress. In week five of her pregnancy she experienced breakthrough bleeding, with more coming in week six. In week eight she felt extreme pain in her lower back and she started hemorrhaging. This lasted for five days. Nisha was surprised and thankful she didn't lose her baby.

As you might guess, it was a loud and clear wake-up call for Nisha. The next day she wrote a pregnancy fitness program and she was going to be her own first client. She started thinking about how she was going to be a healthy expectant mom while being a personal trainer with a growing practice. She was done being in denial. She was, above all else, committed to being physically fit and well.

The fitness regime she created and followed felt great. She got really excited about the opportunity to share her prenatal program with other expectant moms. It became really clear that working with pregnant women would be a core piece of her business. She'd be able to relate to her clients and speak from first-hand experience. Many of her business branding questions were getting answered.

## The prime time to be in the best shape of your life

Nisha could clearly contrast the initial weeks of her pregnancy with the later months of her pregnancy and see what a difference a focus on her physical, nutritional, and emotional well-being provided. As she reflected, Nisha's perspective shifted even further. She began thinking that not only is pregnancy a time when you should focus on taking great care of yourself, it is actually the time to be in your *best* physical shape of your life.

Nisha explained that you are often eating more healthily during pregnancy and you have a reason to get strong – so that you can more easily deliver your baby. You want to maximize your fitness levels so when your baby is born, you have loads of energy to deal with sleep deprivation. And, being in shape during your pregnancy helps you get your body back. You have motivational factors, and it's a time when you are more easily able to tune into what your body needs.

The concept of pregnancy as the prime time to get into your best shape ever challenges me, and I am also inspired by the idea. What a paradigm shift. I think many of us use it as a time to "let go" or "loosen the reigns" on fitness a bit. For me, I had thoughts like, "I'm in good shape for a *pregnant* lady." I never – until my conversation with Nisha – thought of it as a time to be in my best shape ever.

Nancy, Nisha, and others shared some important messages in their stories: There is no standard or typical model for pregnancy physical fitness, so choose the model that works best for you. Listen to your body and do what works. Be honest with yourself about how you're feeling about your weight gain and changing body shape, even if this means expressing disappointment, shame, or frustration. When you're honest with yourself, you can choose the mindset that is truly going to empower you. Perhaps most importantly: Don't compare yourself to or compete with other women! These women's experiences add up to some good advice that is relevant no matter what workout path you declare works best for you.

Check in. What type of workouts do you believe will ideally be best for you?

What mindsets or mantras do you want to keep in mind as you're working out your workouts (or not working out)?

## ❀ OKAY, LET'S BE REAL... ❀ ❀ ❀ ❀ ❀ ❀ ❀ ❀

### Letting go and loving it!

We can feel a lot of pressure from media and from ourselves to stay in shape, be fit, be beautiful. For some of us, the constant assessment of ourselves never stops. There is an incessant voice in our heads that's telling us to get to the gym, or to not eat that piece of cake, or that we must go get highlights or a pedicure. It can get more than a little tiring.

And, let's be real. Pregnancy may be the time you were looking forward to giving yourself a break from all that! After all, you're *supposed* to gain weight and eat for two when you're pregnant! If keeping up with the glitz and glam is stressful or feels inappropriate, then chuck it. During pregnancy, you may choose to focus more on being a mama, than a hot mama. That's totally fine.

Let go and love it. Take a much-deserved break from the judgemental image-assessor in your head. It'd be delightful to turn that part of the brain off for a while and simply love being an expectant mom.

## Appreciating your pregnant body's accomplishments

Adjusting to and accepting your changing body shape, focusing on the changes you most enjoy, determining the clothes styles and fabrics that work best for you, figuring out how to best demonstrate your personal style during pregnancy, and determining the level of physical activity you most desire can feel like a lot of work. For some it is. And there is, at the same time, an opportunity to appreciate all the miraculous accomplishments your pregnant body is achieving.

Each time Diane was pregnant, she marveled at the miracles taking place inside of her. She loved that her body was capable of nourishing a little being who was rapidly developing organs! She took time during each pregnancy to reflect and fully feel the awe of what was taking place. Staying present to the miracles going on in her body helped her keep a healthy perspective about other less desirable aspects of the experience like her hips seemingly getting wider and bigger with each subsequent pregnancy. It kept her focused on the bigger picture and the lovely expansion of her family. She loved what her body was capable of doing!

Dori was a person who was well-endowed in the breast area and as she'd describe, "not particularly perky." She had "gently tolerated" her boobs in the past, yet she felt that perspective shifting for her in a big way as she moved into her second pregnancy.

After her first pregnancy and months of breast feeding, Dori said her breasts were "more objectively absurd than ever." During her second pregnancy when the size started increasing again, she didn't lament the changes or wish them away. Instead, she loved her breasts. Why? Because they showed their worth and they were getting ready to do so again. She had a reason to celebrate them. They nourished and nurtured her child. They had – in Dori's eyes – a critically important function. Before that, it seemed like they were supposed to be entertaining. Now, she had respect for them. Through the process of pregnancy and breast feeding, Dori got a part of her body back.

When Ellen got pregnant, she felt the burden of what was going to be needed physically during her pregnancy. She assumed she would gain a bunch of weight, potentially get stretch marks, be tired, and risk potential surgery during the delivery process – just to name some of the biggies. She clearly knew that physically, she wouldn't come out of this journey the way she went into it. She got herself pretty worked up about all the sacrifices she'd be making with her body and was thinking that her husband had better praise her day and night for what she was doing!

Ellen admitted she'd gotten the martyr act down pretty well. She knew it wasn't good to be feeling like she was making a "whole body" sacrifice day after day. Yet, she didn't know how to shift her thinking.

Then one day Ellen thought she felt her baby move. She tuned in and indeed she felt little flips in her belly. Ellen was profoundly moved by the fact that her body was capable of housing and nourishing a little being who was learning to move inside of her. She was sharing literal space and nutrients with her son or daughter, and it felt like a miracle. The world shifted in that moment, and Ellen was able to tune into her body's accomplishments and capabilities. Her body knew how to prepare for pregnancy and later, for birth. It would know when to go into labor, how to have contractions, how to dilate and stretch and make it possible for her to push a baby out. Ellen found many reasons to appreciate her body, when she started to really zero in on what her body had and would handle successfully.

This doesn't mean that Ellen stopped lamenting about some of the physical changes she endured during pregnancy. She still wasn't thrilled with all her responsibilities as birth mom. She was – however – done being a martyr. She didn't need daily acknowledgement from her husband, about what she was physically doing. She felt lucky and appreciated what she and her body were accomplishing each day.

Check in. What do you appreciate about your pregnant body?

What privileges do you experience in a pregnant body that you can't experience at any other time?

## ❀ Loving How You Look

It is possible to love how you look during pregnancy, and it's okay to *want* to love how you look. You have the opportunity to intentionally choose the image you want to project during pregnancy. Yes, you're the mother of an unborn baby and your body will be shifting to handle that, *and* you can also be the beautiful, sexy, fashionable, and/or fit being you've always been.

To love how you look, remember:

* Focus on what is working for you physically (instead of what isn't).

* Proactively consider how you're going to respond when your body changes and changes in unpredictable ways.

* Avoid comparing your body to others.

* Take the effort to learn your pregnancy shape and what styles and fabrics work best for you.

* Strike a balance that feels great to you for having a fabulous maternity wardrobe and not spending more money than desirable.

* Own and embrace the attention and compliments you get.

* Your body can simultaneously be utilitarian *and* sexy.

* Listen to your body and discover the level of physical exercise and the fitness mindsets that work best for you.

* Appreciate the miraculous achievements of your pregnant body.

Check In. What are the approaches and mindsets that will enable you to love how you look during your pregnancy?

# Facing Your Concerns

I'm actually a bit surprised this book has a chapter entitled, *Facing Your Concerns*. It's a complaint of mine that so many pregnancy resources focus solely on what can go wrong throughout pregnancy. And, in my first pregnancy, I was extremely focused on not getting exposed to any "new" concerns that I hadn't previously known about and didn't subsequently want to worry about. Yet, importantly, I also wanted this book to be authentic and reflect the actualities of pregnancy. And, the reality is that we have concerns when we're expecting. Mine may, of course, vary drastically from yours, yet, we both still have them. You may not have any more concerns during pregnancy than you do at any other time in your life, however, they are likely to be different. So, for these reasons, this chapter was eventually written.

As you step into a pregnancy, there can be an array of concerns that come up. This is understandable. Anxieties can range from uncertainty about which car seat is best to feeling like you don't know how to be a good mother to dealing with the possible discomforts of pregnancy and everything in between. Having concerns is a natural and normal part of being pregnant.

When you commit to loving your pregnant self to the best of your ability, you may feel this means you need to be concern-free. Well, that's just not realistic. You can have concerns and still love the pregnant you. The commitment is precisely what helps bring any worries you might have to the forefront so you can address them. They are an opportunity to discover what is best aligned with who you are and how you want to be as a pregnant person. If you allow yourself to admit and accept the things you are struggling with, they can guide you to important insights about yourself and ultimately show you the choices that best serve you.

Some concerns will take longer than others to decipher, understand, and address. You may have some that are with you for the full length of your pregnancy, never fully receding, even as you create ways to deal with them. Of course, facing an ongoing concern is much different than wallowing. When you wallow, you stay in a state of only seeing and focusing on the problem. You also get into wallowing when you focus solely on what's awful or could be awful without considering why you have the anxiety and how you might deal with it. When you wallow, you further engrain catastrophe thinking and you get "stuck" with the concern. That's not helpful to anyone.

Instead, you want to take a good, thorough, productive look at your concerns so that you can see exactly what you're dealing with and powerfully determine how you want to move forward. You want to examine the concern and fully understand what you are dreading, and not stop there. Keep moving into the realm of: "Okay, this is how I'm currently thinking and feeling about this. How do I want to shift my thoughts and feelings?"

It's also important to mention that *all* concerns are valid. It may seem foolish or "wrong" to be worked up about the size of your thighs when the pregnant woman down the street is on full bed rest and terrified of going into premature labor. You may feel like you should have it more together emotionally as you cry uncontrollably after watching a commercial or receiving a seemingly small piece of bad news. Not necessarily so. Concerns, even those you feel silly about having, are valid. Look at them and find a way to handle the concern, not just shove it aside. You probably know when you're dealing with something in a healthy, straight-forward fashion and when you're avoiding or being passive-aggressive with yourself. And if you don't, you can learn to recognize it with an honest look at yourself.

So, it's not about banishing or avoiding all concerns. It's about looking at your worries in a balanced, healthy way and asking yourself some reflective and forward-focused questions: "What is the crux of your concern? What do you want to do about it? What's possible? In the face of your concern, what empowering mindset can you take on?"

Let's look at how women have dealt with these issues. The specific examples addressed in this chapter may or may not be the same concerns you're currently experiencing or will experience at some point in your pregnancy. This chapter is designed to provide general guidance about facing concerns, rather than prescriptions for facing specific sets of circumstances. If you're not anxious about the same things the women discussed in this chapter were anxious about, then that's great. No need to take on additional worries, that's not the point of this chapter! This chapter is about how you can powerfully handle the concerns you do have, so look at the lessons shared and consider how you might apply them to your situation. And, I'd advise that if reading about a woman's specific worry is making you feel nervous about experiencing the same, go ahead and skip to the next section. Follow your intuition and be on the lookout for what is empowering you and what is not.

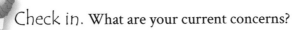

Check in. What are your current concerns?

Which concerns seem the biggest?

Which concerns do you feel like you shouldn't have?

# Different concerns require different approaches

When you have an unclear or unaddressed concern, or many of them, you can easily begin to feel overwhelmed or hopeless. Denise felt this way as she entered her fourth pregnancy. Like many women, she had a range of concerns, and they were exacerbated by the situation surrounding this pregnancy. Denise was serving as a surrogate for a gay couple. Most of you reading this will probably not be considering surrogacy. Yet we all have concerns about pregnancy, and some of yours will likely be similar to Denise's. I think we can all learn from Denise's story.

When you're pregnant, it can be easy to get worried about other people's reactions to what you're doing. When you're pregnant with someone else's baby, it can be *really* easy to get worried about other people's reactions...especially when you have your own questions or doubts about how to best navigate the process. Denise found herself continually apprehensive about what others would think about her choice to be a surrogate, especially because she decided to be a surrogate for a gay couple.

She also had, understandably, uneasy feelings about a number of other aspects of the "being pregnant with someone else's baby" scenario. One was body concerns. How would it feel to have the parents in the delivery room potentially seeing parts of her anatomy that are for "husband's eyes only"?! How much information would they want throughout the pregnancy about her weight gain and measurements and physical condition? How much would she feel comfortable sharing?

Another set of concerns had to do with making sure her immediate family was getting what it needed throughout this process. She didn't want to be any less of a mother. She was anxious that being a surrogate might be asking too much from her family.

Finally, she was nervous about the health of the baby. She had a couple relying on her to nurture their baby sufficiently, lovingly. Denise admitted that she was concerned about the health of this baby more so than her own children; she felt more responsibility.

How did Denise deal with these individual concerns, which seemed overpowering when taken in totality? She had a simple response. "One at a time." Let's learn from her experience.

## Concerning ourselves with what others think

In general, it's a futile endeavor to try to control what other people think. When the topic is out of the mainstream, like surrogacy, the range of reactions is even wider. Denise was cognizant that many people wouldn't know how to respond to the idea of surrogacy, so she would vary how much she shared depending on how well she knew her audience or what the situation was. In situations where she didn't have time to adequately explain, she simply let people believe that she was pregnant with her own baby. With those she knew better, she told them that she was a surrogate. And among those she was feeling most comfortable with in the moment, she'd share the full details.

You may not be dealing with the unique circumstances of a surrogacy, however you can still learn from what Denise did. She didn't want to put herself in the situation where she'd have to wonder, "What are they thinking about me and my choices?" She chose to sidestep it whenever possible. Her example shows us we don't have to provide all the information or put ourselves out there for possible criticism.

For some of us, however, this might not feel like the best approach or even be possible in some circumstances.

Jen did something different. She let her friends and family know when she was open to input and when she was not. She often said something like, "This is not up for discussion. We've decided to look at a couple of daycares in the city. We're excited about what we've seen so far and think this will work great for our family." Then she'd move on. She knew, in her heart of hearts, that she felt good about how she was addressing her childcare-related anxiety. She didn't want others' potentially negative or questioning comments to change her feelings in any way.

Other people may not find your methods to be as enlightened and perfect as you do. You are not always going to get encouraging and enthusiastic responses. Know this. You can ask others to not share their thoughts and opinions. Or, you can decide to not be rattled by what they have to say. Or, at times, you might hear something you were not meant to hear and be able to take it as an opportunity to re-evaluate and recommit to your original choice or make a new one.

The bottom-line is that you want to make choices that result in *you* feeling good, not ones that are designed to appease others or get them to agree with you.

Check In. In what ways are you worried about what others think? What are you worried others will judge you about?

## Nervous about exposure

As her pregnancy continued, Denise grew concerned about exposing her body to and sharing information about the condition of her body with the couple for whom she was a surrogate. She drew on past experience to alleviate this concern. She knew what was discussed at a regular OB-GYN visit. She spent a little time before her first doctor's appointment and determined the level of information she was going to share with the parents afterwards. She decided to go "light" with the information shared and see if they had further questions. This approach worked well. They didn't have much in terms of additional questions, and Denise and the couple quickly found their communication rhythm.

Regardless of your circumstances, there may be physical aspects you don't feel comfortable talking about with your doctor, midwife, your mother, or other people in your life. Again, it's normal to feel uncomfortable. I remember being embarrassed that I was red and itchy "down there" early on during my second pregnancy. It was just extra yeast production and something I'm sure my doctor had seen dozens of times, yet my discomfiture was real. I simply got clear that my desire to get relief and know everything was okay was stronger than my concern about being embarrassed about talking about it.

Denise also knew how a delivery room was set up, and she used that information to ruminate about the delivery room situation. She immediately was clear that she wanted the parents of the baby to be present for the birth. It was then about how to make arrangements and requests that felt most comfortable for her. In the end, it was pretty simple. She asked them to stand near her, up by her head. The parents readily agreed.

It would've been easy for Denise to stay in a place of "This is going to be so uncomfortable to have them see me half naked!" I like how Denise used what she knew to get what she ultimately wanted. Her approach did not mean the concern went away completely, yet, by getting clear that she wanted the parents to experience the birth, that allowed her to say, "Okay, let's stop lamenting about that. They are going to be there, so let's just figure out how."

The fact that we are at least half naked when our babies are born may be unnerving and uncomfortable. I've heard numerous women say that by the end of the pregnancy, they had gotten so used to exposing their belly, having people touch them, having their cervix checked that in the midst of labor and delivery it doesn't occur to them to be concerned. And for some, this is a major shift in accepting or dealing with vulnerability.

The opportunity here is to choose how you're going to relate to your exposure and nudity. Are you going to be fixated on how awful and embarrassing it will be? Or will you look at what's important to you and make any requests or arrangements that you know will make you feel most comfortable? You could, for example, ask your midwife to not use terms or phrases that make you uncomfortable, tell your mom that she cannot come to your check up appointment with you, arrange a home birth with only the people you choose present, ask your doula to help you limit the number of people in the delivery room, tell the hospital staff that you do not want a mirror down there, and any other number of options. And, you could choose to let the rest go.

Check In. What requests do you have to increase your comfort level as you experience increased "exposure" during pregnancy?

## Feeling responsible for the health of the baby

Feeling responsible for the health of the baby was a tough one for Denise. It didn't completely consume her, yet it didn't dissipate, either. And all there was to do about it was to take care of herself and remember that her choices during her first three pregnancies resulted in three healthy babies. There was no reason to assume that anything would be different this time around. And along the way, with each ultrasound where everything looked healthy and right on track, she allowed the concern to weaken.

It's easy for pregnant women to put pressure on themselves about making sure their babies are healthy and are getting the best possible experience inside of the womb. Many women think, "I've got to do everything I can and everything absolutely right for those nine months." And it can be easy to think that any bump in the road is your fault. Right? The baby is inside of your body and you are in charge of the environment. It can add up to a lot of pressure.

Do you want to listen to your body and make intentional choices about what to eat and drink and how to move your body? Sure. Do you want to become consumed and fill your life with absolute "must dos" and "must not haves?" No. You want to strike the balance between the two that works for you. For some people, a little extra pressure on themselves helps them perform and behave in the most advantageous way. Others know that they thrive when they kick back and adopt the "everything in moderation" philosophy. You've got to find *your* equilibrium.

I acknowledge that some of you will deal with important health concerns for your babies that are not easily dismissed, diminished, or addressed. I've spoken with women, like Tamara, who had a history of birth defects in her family and women over 44, like Jennifer, who were terrified of having babies with chromosome irregularities. These types of concerns are not easy to set aside. Yet, Tamara and Jennifer did, at times, find ways to do so.

Tamara clearly realized that her fear was not going to do her or her baby any good. For her, it was a matter of putting her faith in God. She knew that she could make healthy choices for herself and she realized that was all she could do. The rest was not in her control. She gave up trying to hold the reins. Jennifer constantly reminded herself of her belief that she could handle whatever was given her. She always had and she knew she always would. This belief kept her calm and focused on what she could do, rather than worrying about what *might* happen.

Check In. What thoughts will support you to be a health-conscious (and not a health-obsessed) expectant mother?

## Being less available for others

Denise's concerns about being less available for her family or having them suffer in any way due to her commitment to this other family was one that she struggled with throughout her pregnancy. She had pretty consistent worries about how her family might be affected when she spent time talking with the baby's parents, when she went to doctor's appointments, when she needed extra rest, or when she simply sat and rubbed her belly spending time with and loving the baby. She felt there were no easy answers about how to be there for everyone, in the ways she ideally wanted, during the nine months of her pregnancy.

It can be a common theme during pregnancy. How do you find the time to nourish yourself, take good care of your developing baby, and fulfill your responsibilities to all the others in your life like you have in the past?

For Denise, the concern about being there less for others helped her be intentional about the ways in which she was choosing to spend her time. For example, when she stopped to put her feet up when she got home at the end of the day, she'd ask herself: "Is there something I feel is important to do with or for my family right now that I want to be doing instead of resting?" Sometimes the answer was "Yes;" her daughter had a school project due the next day or she could tell that her husband had a hard day and needed to talk. Often the answer was "No;" immediate needs were taken care of or could be handled after dinner and she could allow herself to set her guilt aside.

Denise made headway with releasing this concern, yet it never fully went away. That's an important point. Not all concerns go away or become negligible. The goal here is *not* to go for a perfect history of noticing, fully addressing, and erasing all concerns all the time. Often, it's a messy, non-linear process where concerns will resurface even after you believe you've "handled" them.

I hope that you're embracing the idea that it's okay, and even useful, to have concerns. By experiencing them, you're given the opportunity to address them and take new actions or think new thoughts that are better lined up with how you want to be as a pregnant person. This can be a very empowering perspective. The next question that might come up is, "I know I have the opportunity to address a concern. That's useful. But, *how* do I address it? How do I handle it or minimize it most effectively?"

# Deal with your concerns powerfully

When you become aware of a concern, it can help to ask yourself two layers of questions.

First, identify your concern and then look at it a little deeper. Ask yourself "What are you *really* worried about?" Your concern might appear to be one thing, but, in actuality it's about something else under the surface.

For instance, if you find yourself overly obsessed with thinking about the health of your baby, dig a little deeper. What are your specific worries? Is it that you have a hereditary disease that you're afraid your baby will get? That you will use pregnancy as an excuse to not be as physically active as you want to be? That giving up or scaling back on caffeine for the health of your baby is a lifestyle change you wish you didn't have to make because you'll miss your daily coffee fix?

What are the anxious feelings specifically pointing to? You can dig in and create some clarity around what vague, yucky feelings are telling you. To do this you could try talking about your feelings with a trusted friend or coach, or journaling about what you're experiencing. You could spend some time answering the How, What, Where, and When questions: How do I feel? What thoughts trigger the feelings? When did I start feeling this way? Where – in what circumstances and where in your body – do you feel the anxious feelings? Another powerful question is: "If I had a magic wand, what would I ideally like to have happen?" By taking a closer look you can determine what, precisely, your concern is and why you are experiencing it.

Next, ask yourself, "What can I do about it?" Once you're clear about what specifically is bothering you, courses of action might come immediately to mind. Or, you may want to sit down and brainstorm with yourself or a friend on how you could take a positive step to deal with the issue. You could also look online for ideas or look to related (or even unrelated) stories in this book and other pregnancy resources for ideas. You may find that there are indeed many options to consider. If so, you want to look at what best resonates for you. What is going to alleviate the specific concern you just dissected?

For instance, if you're afraid your daughter will get a hereditary disease that your mom had, there are a number of things you could do. You could research the topic or ask your doctor about it or decide that it is out of your control and choose to let it go.

If you're concerned that you're using pregnancy as an excuse to be less physically active, then you could choose to get a prenatal fitness coach or ask a friend to take a walk with you every morning or make some other commitment that you feel is best for you and your baby.

The bottom line is to understand your concern and specifically ask yourself what, if anything, you want to do about it. It may take just a moment to get clear about your concern and decide what you want to do, and it may be an inquiry and series of exercises that take much longer or that you revisit over time. You'll need to pay attention to your intuition to determine what's most appropriate and know when you're ready to take action and move on.

The key is to not ignore your anxious or worrisome feelings. Look at them at a deeper level and determine if there's anything to do. Sometimes what you do about a concern is simply decide to let it go or accept that things are as they are. Trust yourself. Only you can know if you're engaging with your concerns in a constructive, healthy manner.

As Denise continued to explore her concern about not being available enough for her family during surrogacy, she learned a valuable lesson. For her, the anxious feelings were pointing to an ongoing desire to balance her needs with her family's needs. She realized it wasn't a concern that was unique during her pregnancy; it was simply exacerbated during her pregnancy. She assumed that since she was going to need to take more time for herself, the time spent with her family would consequently decline. And since this pregnancy wasn't *for* her family, she worried they would resent the time and attention she focused elsewhere. After she pinpointed the root of the problem, Denise clearly saw that she needed to have a conversation with her husband and children to let them know that she was aware of and concerned about the impact her pregnancy would have on them. An important conversation ensued and Denise emerged feeling fully loved and supported by her family.

Denise took a closer look at what was causing her anxious feelings and realized what she was most distressed about. Knowing this clearly, she then could see the action that would be most likely to alleviate these feelings. Taking these steps went a long way towards minimizing Denise's pregnancy-enhanced concern.

Check in. What is your biggest concern?

What is this particular concern pointing to? What are you *really* concerned about?

What is there to do about this concern to help alleviate your anxiety?

## ✿ OKAY, LET'S BE REAL...

Don't give me more concerns!

Yes, being worried about pregnancy and childbirth is normal and natural. And yes, all concerns are valid. And, yes, concerns fulfill a useful purpose as they help us uncover what's most important to us.

But, no, we do *not* need other people, magazine articles, television shows, websites, or even pregnancy books (!) dishing up concerns to us that we hadn't even thought of yet!

When we tell people our birth plans, we don't want them telling us to be on the lookout for the litany of problems they know laboring moms have faced in the past. When we're researching how to deal with X, it's not useful to be asked if we've thought about Y (where Y= an even bigger potential problem).

We already have enough concerns. We don't need new ones!

Of course, we could simply decide to not take on new concerns. We can turn the page, change the channel, close the website, and ask people to not tell us horror stories. We can choose to continue with the mindsets we established for ourselves. Yet, it would sure help us a great deal and save us some time, if we weren't presented with "new" concerns to consider.

# Physical challenges

What if the concerns we're grappling with are not in our minds? What if we have a real physical ailment or challenge that we're dealing with?

Our bodies are taking on a miraculous task. All the intricately integrated pieces that are flowing together synchronously and sequentially to create a life boggles my mind and puts me in a place of complete awe. And, since there's a lot going on in our pregnant bodies, there will be different physical sensations that we'll experience.

Physical changes are taking place and, as a result, physical challenges of different sorts can crop up during a pregnancy. Examples could include fatigue, morning sickness, hip discomfort, restless energy, and acid reflux.

I asked women about how they dealt physically, emotionally, and mentally with physical discomfort or pain. The theme I heard over and over again, in different variations, was that while you might not be able to control what happens to you physically (although you certainly influence this), you can control how you respond to what happens. You can be aware of your thinking and make adjustments when your thoughts don't serve you. And ultimately when you make shifts in your thinking, it can shift the way you feel.

Betsy, who experienced a few of the aforementioned symptoms, took the approach that you don't need to know ahead of time how you'll deal with specific physical ailments. She said this for a couple of reasons. First, you don't know if you'll even experience them. She advised against reading resources that tell you about all the unwanted symptoms you might possibly experience during pregnancy. There's no point in getting worked up about something that might not happen! Second, when you do experience something that needs to be addressed, there are plenty of resources out there, including the great people in your life, to reference and give you ideas about how to best move forward. Betsy pointed out that when you're actually experiencing discomfort, that's when your instincts kick in real-time and enable you to determine the best approach for you.

She also had a great approach to the changes her body was going through during her pregnancy. She knew there might be times when she'd need more sleep, or have to alter her exercise regime or make some other change to her routine. She intentionally chose to think about them as "adjustments" and not as "limitations" or "burdens." She determined early on how she wanted to approach whatever physical changes occurred without concerning herself with specifics that might or might not happen. And whatever was going to pop up for her, she had a plan to keep an open and positive mindset about them.

Check In. How do you want to approach the physical adjustments you'll experience?

It's well-known that there are physical ailments that are considered "common" during pregnancy. Morning sickness, fatigue, swollen ankles, back pain, and shortness of breath, to name a few. While many pregnant women experience these, I want to share the idea that you don't *have* to get these ailments. You don't *need* to expect to experience them. It's not a "given," even if a condition is hereditary. It may be a well-known fact that women in your family retain water and swell during pregnancy. You may have been told for years that you can look forward to this phenomenon. You might be the exception.

Also, it doesn't have to go exactly the way it did in your last pregnancy. Certainly, if you experienced back pain in your first pregnancy, it might mean that it's more likely to occur again in your second. Yet, I'd encourage you to question the idea that it *has* to happen again. Sure, you may have received what seems like irrefutable medical information, yet there are also new remedies, approaches, and ideas conceived every day. Also, you will have different experiences in each pregnancy. Many mothers of two or more can attest to this. Instead of defaulting to "I'll have to endure that again" or "I'll be really tired throughout my first trimester because that's what happened before" or "I'm not looking forward to retaining water," the belief we can hold on to is actually that no two pregnancies are alike.

Heidi, for example, had four different pregnancies and they had been just that… different. With her first child, she felt nauseous a good deal of the time. She had swelling and low energy levels, feeling tired throughout the pregnancy. In her second pregnancy, she felt sick again and experienced spotting, cramping, swollen legs and arms, and preterm labor. After those experiences, you might think that she was resigned to life being pretty miserable as a pregnant person.

Yet, this wasn't the case for Heidi. She attributed her physical struggles to the fear and anxiety she felt during her first two pregnancies. This was empowering to Heidi. She didn't have a physical condition that was unalterable or insurmountable. Instead, she believed that if she could find the means to reduce the stress and anxiety that she felt, then she could experience something different physically. This allowed Heidi to embark on her next pregnancy with a much different approach.

With her third pregnancy, Heidi was "ready" in all senses of the word. She knew she could create a different journey, and she did. She did everything her midwife told her to do. She exercised, took calcium, vitamin B, prenatal vitamins, and ate really well.

She believed that she'd find remedies that would work for her even though she hadn't in the past. When she started feeling nauseous, she ordered a tummy-soothing product online, and she felt better immediately. She also found relief from smelling peppermint oil. Her approach and attitude were lighter – more playful and exploratory – and her pregnancy was much more enjoyable.

A couple things are important about Heidi's story. One, she had vastly different experiences during her pregnancies. And mentally, she did not get locked into thinking that her pregnancy was going to feel a certain way. She didn't get stuck believing that she was destined to feel bad in all her pregnancies. At the same time, she didn't feel like she did it "wrong" in her first two pregnancies. Instead, she accepted that her experiences might vary.

Remember, your attitude makes a difference in how you feel physically. If you feel you're doomed to experience a litany of problems, then you are, in essence, programming your mind and body to be on the lookout for problems or for problematic symptoms. Then when any little glitch or shift occurs, you're ready to think, "Yup, there it is. There's a problem I knew was coming!"

When you're *not* resigned to the idea that you'll have to suffer, a shift or a new kind of physical symptom doesn't make you leap to the assumption that it'll lead to big problems. Instead, you open yourself up to all kinds of possibilities. You can think, "Oh, this is different. What is this? And what can I do about it?" You might actually try a nausea remedy you see advertised online because you're not resigned to the idea that you'll have morning sickness and there's nothing you can do about it.

When you stay aware about what assumptions you are making, it will have an impact on how you experience, respond to, and treat the physical shifts you encounter. Remember that your thoughts and feelings have an impact on your physical well-being. I'm not saying that you can magically think your physical symptoms away. Yet, it's important to acknowledge that your mental, emotional, and physical well-being are interconnected.

Check in. What thoughts and beliefs do you have that impact your physical well-being in a positive way?

What thoughts and beliefs do you have that might impact your physical well-being in a negative way?

## When it doesn't go according to plan

It can be empowering and useful to expect and plan for your pregnancy experience to go smoothly. It is helpful to not be on the lookout for problems and invite them in. So what if you're taking this approach and everything doesn't fall in line with your "smooth and easy" plan?

Even when you have very real and intrusive physical symptoms to deal with, your thoughts and attitude will impact the level of ease or difficulty you experience related to your physical symptoms.

For Leslie, her pregnancy experience was about reacting to what came up more than having a specific plan about how everything was going to come together. She had ideas about how she'd like things to go and she said, "I did recognize that you can make a great plan, but you had better be prepared for the plan to fall off the rails." This was useful self-coaching for Leslie when it came to dealing with her and her babies' health during her pregnancies, as she was thrown some curve balls.

In her first pregnancy, Leslie had the unique challenge of cholestasis. Cholestasis occurs when your liver does not eliminate bile acids effectively and they build up in your bloodstream. It makes you itchy, really itchy. Your skin also can take on a yellowish hue. Of course, it had not been in Leslie's plans to deal with extreme discomfort or people's strange looks or questions about her coloring. She could've easily spent the months she had cholestasis lamenting about how awful her experience was (and she could've gotten a lot of agreement about that, I'm sure.) Instead, Leslie handled it head on. She knew she had it, she knew she was doing all she could to alleviate it, and she knew it had to run its course. So, she was straight-forward with herself and with others. She told people what was going on so she didn't feel the need to pretend she wasn't itchy or hope they wouldn't notice her coloring was a little off.

In both her pregnancies, Leslie had gestational diabetes. With this diagnosis there were specific things she had to do every day to manage her health, including restrictions on what she could eat. There were times she had to leave work meetings so she could give herself an insulin shot. She needed to eat at inconvenient times. It was a nuisance.

This is again where Leslie's self-coaching about going with the flow came in handy.

She told herself there was no point in resisting the inevitable. She could try to ignore it or feel unjustly burdened or think of all the reasons why this shouldn't be happening to her, or she could wrap her head around it and begin to map out the best ways to deal with the circumstances.

Leslie didn't get to choose whether she got cholestasis or gestational diabetes. She did, however, get to choose how she was going to respond and move forward. She decided to get busy dealing with her physical challenges as best she could. She put a fairly quick stop to the lamenting and this allowed her to move on and be able to truly identify the best ways for her to address her diagnosis.

While pregnant with her second, Carla experienced a few things that could lead one to be disgruntled about pregnancy. She had back and neck pain and other discomfort that she hadn't experienced with her first. As someone who had suffered from headaches and migraines in the past, Carla wasn't surprised to have some head pain. Yet, her headaches were more frequent and more painful in her second pregnancy. And, as her pregnancy progressed, her toddler moved into a new phase expressing more independence and no longer going along with routines he had previously enjoyed. She and her husband were struggling to find new ways of operating that worked for the family and the solutions were not immediately evident. (That might sound familiar to many of us who are not pregnant for the first time!) I figured these circumstances would get her down; that she'd be counting her days until her baby was born.

Carla looked at her circumstances differently. For her, she was clear that she chose to have a second child and she knew that women dealt with far worse. She felt there was nothing to do, except to buck up and handle it. She knew it wouldn't last forever. She wanted another child and this was the path to get there. There wasn't any sense in complaining in Carla's mind.

Her answer to many of my questions was, "You just do it." She didn't worry much about how she was going to handle circumstances or how much longer a headache would last or how much worse the back pain might get. She was going to experience it regardless. Sometimes, it can be that simple.

The point is to find the mindset that allows you to look forward and move forward, so that you're not stuck or feeling victimized. So whether it's "Expect the best" or "Okay, how can I handle this my way?" or "Just buck up and do it," find the perspective in circumstances you're in that will enable you to approach them powerfully.

Check In. What mindset or mantra empowers you (or could empower you) to deal with challenges in a powerful way?

# No "should-ing" on yourself

The perspectives that will work for each of us will vary greatly. What doesn't work is when you tell yourself that you "should" do something you don't truly want to do or that you "should" feel a way that you actually don't feel. "Should-ing" on yourself can manufacture concerns where none need exist. You may wish that you wanted to eat a totally organic diet or you may want to feel peaceful when a girlfriend questions a choice you've made. Yet, if you tell yourself you "should" do something that's not aligned with how you truly feel, you'll set yourself up to fall short.

The point here is that you need to do what uniquely works for you. You don't want to "should" on yourself, and rigidly adhere to how things have to be done because it's the norm, because it's what we "should" want, or because things "should" go exactly the same in your second pregnancy as they did in your first. You can create each pregnancy uniquely. That's the magic of it. As your journey unfolds, you get to decide each step along the way and determine what is working for you in this moment, and then in this moment, and this moment, and so on. You can make shifts as you continue along your journey. You are not locked into a decision. You are allowed to change your mind.

Yet, sometimes that is easier said than done. Nancy was pregnant with her second baby when we spoke, and she was struggling with the idea of having another drug-free delivery. She was very proud of what she had accomplished with the birth of her first child. She had always been inspired by other mothers who had given birth naturally, without any drugs, and she wanted to be able to do the same. Part of her reasoning was to avoid any potential side effects of the drugs, yet, more importantly, she wanted to know that she was a strong woman who could give birth naturally.

She accomplished that! She also admitted it was more painful than she had imagined or wanted. Now in her second pregnancy, she was thinking about having an epidural. Her husband was happy to support her in either choice. Yet, Nancy was beating herself up about her change of heart. She kept asking herself, "Why are you even considering it? You know you can do it without it." But, she was also being honest. She was scared and she didn't want to feel that pain again. As grateful as she was for the experience the first time, she was not eager to repeat it.

Nancy's was a tricky situation. Would it be a relief to simply allow herself to get the epidural and not worry about the pain? Or would it feel better to work on setting her fears aside so she could experience another natural childbirth and feel empowered by her achievement? Only Nancy could answer those questions.

Here is what I'd like to offer to all of us when we're faced with a similar situation where neither choice feels 100 percent good and we're concerned about our decision.

## What to consider when both the choices concern you

If one of the choices doesn't feel good because it seemingly flies in the face of what you've said or done in the past, remember we can always choose to do something different. And, that doesn't negate or invalidate what we did previously. If Nancy chose to have an epidural with her second baby, it wouldn't change the convictions she had when she chose the natural route the first time. It doesn't mean she's contradicting herself, or that she was wrong one time and right the other. The choice can be "right" in both situations. It is possible for us to choose two different things at two different times and have both choices be in alignment with our values and who we are.

You can also change your mind midstream. You are not locked into your choice forever. Your thinking may shift in the coming weeks and cause you to choose again and choose differently. I think it's quite powerful and empowering when someone confidently owns her decision to change course. Yes, people might question the change. You can choose to be okay with that, too. You can say, "Yup, I changed my mind. Here's what I discovered to be even more critical for myself..."

As you're deliberating, it's also important to remember that there are almost always more than just two choices. It could seem clear that Nancy's choices are to give birth naturally or to have an epidural, yet there are variations. She could decide to go natural unless labor lasts more than a certain number of hours, consider narcotic assistance that's not an epidural, or wait until labor starts and see what her intuition tells her then. There are a variety of ways you can approach the decisions you make.

It's common to feel like you "should" do something a certain way because that's what you've done in the past or that's what people would expect of you or that's what you've been telling yourself you want to do. Instead, you can freely choose what you want in that moment. It's okay to change your mind, it's possible to make up your own unique way of approaching an issue, and it might even be best to decide to not decide.

Often, when none of the choices are feeling good, it's best to not make a choice. Just stay in the stage of contemplation. You don't have to force a decision like we sometimes feel pressured to do. You can give yourself the time and space to say to yourself and to others that you don't know yet, you're still deciding. You want to feel confident and empowered about your choice and you can take the time you need to get to that space. This approach does not represent a person who doesn't know her mind or her convictions. It's a person who is in integrity and alignment with what she says she's committed to.

Check in. Where are you "should-ing" on yourself?

What choice would actually feel best to you?

## Push your boundaries

As we've discussed, there isn't just one way to be pregnant. You have the opportunity to listen to your internal voices, trust your intuition, and discover your own way of being pregnant.

Naoli is a midwife and she talked of the amazing depth of maternal instinct that we all have that gets ignited during pregnancy. She believes it's most useful for pregnant women to expose themselves to a wide range of advice and then apply only what feels useful. She says that we know best, even better than medical professionals, about what is going to work and feel good for us.

Naoli practiced what she preaches during her pregnancy and completely set aside her concerns of what others might think! She, for example, gave herself permission to fall asleep during a meeting at work. Everyone was gathered around the conference table and she was feeling extremely tired, so she simply and unapologetically allowed herself to go to sleep at the table. She unabashedly allowed herself to take what she needed in that moment regardless of what others, including herself, might think about it.

Undoubtedly, falling asleep in a work meeting might be well beyond your comfort zone or what you consider to be acceptable behavior. I'd be with you on that. I share Naoli's story to challenge you to stretch your boundaries.

Sometimes, what feels best goes against societal norms or what are the expected or assumed choices. This can be a tough one. It's common to be fearful of the judgment that comes with doing something that is unexpected or that might not present us as 100 percent fully competent super woman every moment of every day. That is why pregnancy is an opportunity to increase your capacity to not concern yourself with the opinions of others.

Set your concerns aside and make sure you're giving yourself full permission to follow your intuition in the moment, even if your instincts are pointing towards something whimsical or unexpected or seemingly inappropriate.

Check In. In what ways can you push your boundaries? What could you audaciously give yourself permission to do?

## You're doing it your way

Lettie made a choice that others might judge negatively. During her second trimester, she hosted Thanksgiving for more than 20 family members while her husband was in the hospital, and she had just moved into her house three weeks earlier.

While most would see that choice as an incredible burden, Lettie wanted, in that space and time, to celebrate with her loved ones. She had put in a lot of time and effort to make her vision of the holiday possible. On Thanksgiving Day, she suspected that she might crash once everyone had gone home, yet during that evening, she felt the pride that accompanied such a task. It had looked insurmountable earlier in the week and some of her family members were concerned that she was overdoing it. Yet, Lettie had somehow known that she would get it done and she felt so much peace in the moment. As she reflected, she realized that her journey to that day had been filled with moments of peace. She had known she could do it.

The day after Thanksgiving, Lettie did indeed surrender and she sat on her couch for two days. Lettie gave herself permission to take the rest that she needed. Her eight-year-old and six-year-old got their own cereal and watched mom on the couch. By Sunday, she was back in action and participated in prayer and got the emotional hugs she needed to complete her rejuvenation.

It's easy to judge that a pregnant woman shouldn't push herself to a point where she needs two days to recuperate. However, the only one who could say what was right for Lettie was Lettie herself. For her, it felt good to "push" herself to move into their new home and host a big celebration while her husband was in the hospital. That's what brought her the most joy during that time. She didn't want to sit around doing nothing thinking about how long it was taking her husband to recover. She wanted the love and celebration to christen her new home at Thanksgiving. This made her feel good and felt important to her family. At the same time, Lettie knew her efforts took a toll on her. She didn't beat herself up about this. She didn't turn her accomplishment into a failure because she crashed afterwards or because some people didn't agree with her choices.

When Georgia was pregnant she noticed that many women wanted to tell her their labor and delivery stories. Georgia didn't want to hear them. She didn't want to "take on" aspects of other people's deliveries. She wanted to create her own. Now Georgia is a caring, polite person, and it felt uncomfortable for her to stop the conversation when women started sharing. And the women themselves seemed surprised or shut down by her request to wait to tell her their stories about delivery until *after* she experienced her own delivery. I can imagine being geared up to share my personal story and feeling let down or even annoyed that someone wasn't willing to listen. I applaud Georgia's intentionality and willingness to make the "tell me later" request repeatedly even though it would potentially frustrate others (and even though it would've meant that she wouldn't want to read sections of this book until after her delivery!).

There are unique decisions you may make that may trigger others to feel annoyed, uncomfortable, disappointed, or even concerned for you. This doesn't mean that the choice is wrong. That's not to say you shouldn't take into consideration the impact of your decision on others. Your significant other (or the baby's father), especially, is certainly entitled to opinions and requests regarding his unborn baby's care. How he and others think and feel are important parts of determining whether a choice fully works for you. Yet, also know that when you have taken into consideration all that you feel you need to and are unabashedly doing what works for you, people may have strong reactions. Do your best to arrive at what truly resonates for you and accept that what works for you may not work for others.

Check in. In what ways are you being pregnant "your way?"

Where are you conforming to approaches that are not fully your own?

## OKAY, LET'S BE REAL... ✼ ✼ ✼ ✼ ✼ ✼ ✼ ✼

### I haven't a clue!

Let's be frank about something. This philosophy of doing pregnancy your way can sound great in theory and, at times, it can be *so* much easier said than done! You may, in certain circumstances or in certain aspects of your pregnancy, feel utterly clueless.

In some circumstances, it can feel downright impossible to try to figure out what you want, let alone make whatever you want happen. This is fine. Let yourself have no clue.

The time and energy it would take to process your thoughts and feelings to arrive at *your* choice may feel exhausting and overwhelming. You may feel like giving up, or you may just want someone else to choose for you.

If you don't have a clue, then you don't have a clue! Don't force it. Don't feel bad about it. Just let yourself be...clueless. We're totally entitled to that at times.

## Our nasty comparisons

Too often, when women think about how they're doing in life, they don't give themselves credit for progress: how far they've come, what they've achieved, how they've grown, or how they've expanded their capacities. Instead we often take out an imaginary yardstick and only judge ourselves by how we compare to others. As explored in the last chapter, *Loving How Your Look*, it's often not useful to compare, for example, the weight we gain or the speed at which we gain it with others' experiences. We want to let our experience be our experience without having to measure and compare. This applies to other aspects of pregnancy as well. It's too easy to see another person excelling in an aspect of pregnancy and then start to get anxious that we're not doing it right or well enough. We notice and get concerned about this perceived "gap" and totally forget about our accomplishments. I, personally, easily fall victim to these nasty comparisons!

When I consider how I rate at marketing and growing my business, I compare myself to the best business development person I know. When I consider my level of health and well-being, I compare myself to the person who is employed as a personal trainer and runs ultra-marathons. When I consider how I'm doing as a mom, I get so very nasty with myself. I think about the lady who seems so emotionally connected to her children; the mom who plans and executes weekly, home-cooked, organic meals; the mom who is beautifully scrapbooking her pregnancy; the parents who have the nursery all stocked and ready to go; etc. I end up comparing myself to this composite of the perfect woman (like putting together Angelina Jolie's lips, with Gwyneth Paltrow's nose and Jennifer Garner's dimples...). And I can't measure up!

If you fall into this very human and seductive comparison pitfall, you will never win. You'll have anxieties that you don't need to have. There are always going to be women out there who are being more intentional, spending more time, or doing something better in some aspect of mothering. The pressure during pregnancy can be even more intense because it's a concentrated and proscribed period of time. The thinking is often, "You can pull yourself together and get with the program for just nine months out of your life, can't you?"

So, what are you to do about our tendency to make nasty comparisons? How do you continually face your concerns and perceived insufficiencies in an empowering, effective way? Here's what those who have gone before say.

## Let your values guide you

First, understand what's most important to you. What are your values? Is it more important to maintain an all-organic, well-balanced diet or to engage in activities that have you feeling peaceful and grounded? Is it more important to have the kitchen cleaned up and organized or to give yourself an hour of rest? Some of you will choose one; some of you will choose the other. Sometimes, you'll say they both are important. And sometimes your answer might be different than it was the day before. The question is, "Right now, in this moment, what is most important to you, your family, and how you're committed to living?" When you clarify your priorities, then it's easier to resist comparing yourself to others in areas that you've intentionally decided are not areas of focus for you.

Angel knew that a clean and organized house was good for her family. A clean house helped keep her family healthy. And when the house was organized, everyone knew where to find things. With two young kids who often needed something *right now*, it helped to have everything in its place.

Yet, when Angel was pregnant with her third baby, she knew she had to make some choices. She needed more time to rest and take care of herself, and she didn't want to cut back on the time she interacted with her older children. Taking care of herself and playing with her kids became the priority over a neat and organized home. It bugged her at first, not being able to live up to her prior standards, but she let the house go a little bit. It required that she stop comparing herself to how she used to be. It meant that she had to set aside her concerns about not being a good homemaker. Finally, it sometimes even felt liberating! She kept reminding herself of her focus and her choice. She could say to herself, "I could continue to have a perfectly put together house, and I'm choosing to rest or play with my kids instead."

Check in. What's most important to you?

What can you let go of?

A great way to avoid the pitfall of comparing yourself to others is to clearly know what's most important to you and to know that you've made the intentional choice to prioritize based on your values. Being gentle with yourself, not holding yourself to impossibly high standards, and generally giving yourself a break are ways to avoid focusing on short-falls rather than accomplishments.

## Give yourself a break!

As you're pregnant and as you continue to move through the various phases of parenthood, you're going to be consistently doing things you've never done before. You're going to be fielding questions about when you're due, gaining pregnancy weight, preparing for delivery, adjusting to new sleep schedules, receiving opinions about what sorts of childcare work best, determining how you want to handle discipline, and the list goes on and on. These are new endeavors, and it's highly unlikely you're going to be immediately skilled in these areas. You are unfamiliar with what thoughts, feelings, and reactions you'll have, and this may be a source of anxiety for many.

Too often, we expect perfection from ourselves right out of the gate. It's not fair. You wouldn't expect someone to be perfect at tennis the first time he picks up a racket, so why hold yourself to an impossible standard? Give yourself some breaks. You will make mistakes. You will continue to make mistakes as the parenting journey continues and you enter each new phase with your child. The sooner you accept that you'll be messing up along the way, the sooner you can actually see and learn the lessons presented in each set new of circumstances.

When I was pregnant with my second child, I called up my friend Thea in a moment of complete overwhelm. It was near the end of my pregnancy and I was already making post-maternity business commitments. A zillion questions and concerns were running through my head: "What time in the morning can I actually expect to be at a meeting? What kind of sleep schedule will my son be on? How long will it take to get two kids up and ready and dropped off at daycare?" I often felt short of time with just one kid. How was I going to get it all done with two? I spewed this litany of questions at Thea and she chuckled sympathetically and said something along the lines of, "And you expect yourself to be able to answer all these questions today?"

We went on to talk about how you just don't know until you know. All I could do was make my best guesses about how it would work in the future and adjust from there. Thea shared that she didn't know how to be a mother to a three-year-old boy and she didn't know how to pick the best preschool for her son. Yet, she'd soon be doing both. I realized that I needed to adjust to a lifetime of adjusting. And to do that, I was going to have to give myself a break and allow for some imperfections.

## Accept help

Thea also was able to give me some concrete ideas about how to best transition out of maternity leave, as she, too, was an independent business owner. Which leads to the next piece of advice mothers have shared time and again: accept help. This concept is covered in detail in the *Choosing Your Care and Support* chapter, yet I think it also bears repeating here. Too often we have concerns and then when someone offers to support us in some way, we reject the offer! So, accept the help that is offered you and ask for and accept the help you'd like to have. You don't have to wait until you're in a crisis situation to reach out. You could reach out all the time. It doesn't have to mean you're weak or incapable. In fact, it can mean that you're gracious, generous with sharing yourself, and really smart!

You do not need to figure this all out on your own. Yes, you are on a unique and personal journey. Still, you can still get plenty of ideas and inspiration from others. Some of what people offer you will resonate and some won't.

Give yourself full permission to be resourceful. If you're anxious about registering for all the appropriate and best baby products, see how you can lighten your load. If your friend enjoyed registering for baby gifts and is consistently raving about her burp-free bottles and how her diaper bag has pockets in all the right places, take her with you when you register. Or ask for a short list of "must have" items. Or ask her if she'd be willing to handle the complete registry process for you! Look at *who* can help you and *how* they can help you. Where can you skip doing the work because someone already has?

Check In. What can you ask for help with right now?

## Take care of yourself

A final way to take the pressure off and stop comparing yourself to others is to simply take really great care of yourself. Again, this was covered in the *Choosing Your Care and Support* chapter: you can't take care of others, if you don't take care of yourself. You may know this intellectually somewhere in the recesses of your brain, yet women too often neglect to put this wisdom into practice. Especially when we're concerned about something, we may feel that we've got to do something, address the concern in some way, before we could possibly think about nourishing or pampering ourselves. Sometimes when it feels least appropriate is when it's most needed.

Remember, taking care of yourself means physically giving yourself what you crave and nourishing your intellectual or creative curiosity. You may also want to consider ways that you can take care of yourself in the moment, in any moment, no matter where you are. Deep breathing and listening to music are examples. Taking care of yourself can even look like bitching and moaning and getting some empathy from others! Sometimes you just need to get it out!

At any given moment, you can look for the best ways to take care of yourself. It is a practice that takes constant revisiting and is extremely nourishing when you let yourself discover new and interesting ways to augment your self-care.

Check In. What do you know are the most nourishing ways to take care of yourself?

## ❀ Facing Your Concerns

Having concerns is a natural and normal part of being pregnant. All concerns are valid. There's no need to compare your concerns to others' concerns or to dismiss what's got you worried.

It's not about having zero concerns. It's about looking at your worries in a balanced, healthy way and asking yourself some reflective and forward-focused questions.

* Find your equilibrium. Listen to yourself and your body and make intentional choices. Avoid getting consumed and filling up your life with absolute "must dos" and "must nots."

* When you become aware of a concern, it can help to ask yourself: "What am I *really* concerned about?" Follow it with: "What is there to do about it?"

* You may not be able to control all the physical shifts that take place in your body. You can control how you respond to those shifts.

* You are uniquely creating your pregnancy. There is nothing you "should" do. You can do it your way.

* You can change your mind at any time.

* To take pressure off yourself during pregnancy, pick what's most important to you (and let go of the rest), give yourself a break (you've never done this before), accept help, and take care of yourself.

Check In. What, for you, are the keys to powerfully facing your concerns?

# Experiencing the Miracle of Birth

Ah, the birth of your child. It's a monumental, life-altering experience in your life. No matter what you experience – whether your delivery turns out to be easy, difficult, joyful, painful, intensely emotional, highly unpredictable, or a mix of these – it's a unique, personal rite of passage. And, you have an opportunity to identify and discover the type of experience you most want to have.

Determining what *you* want for your delivery experience – and, again, not what others try to influence you to choose or what you think you *should* choose – helps you to plan for and prepare yourself physically and emotionally for the birth process. Your experience may not be what you hoped for. Unexpected things may take place. Yet, by understanding the options that truly resonate for you, you are much more likely to take actions and adopt perspectives that can help you create what you want and that can help you no matter how things go.

## What do you want for your birth experience?

So, what do you want your childbirth experience to be like? What's important to you? There are many ways to consider this question. Is it to be pain-free? Is it to feel your son or daughter being born? Is it to share an intimate experience with your significant other? Is it to share the experience with as many as possible? Is it to be in tune with your body? Is it most important to you to feel connected with your baby? And, where do you want to give birth? How do you want to feel during the process? How do you want to feel about yourself as you bring a baby into the world? What is it that you want to focus on?

To gain clarity on what you want, start with the most prevalent questions that are in your head. Your questions might be: "How long will delivery take? What will it feel like? What will be my reaction to pain and each step of the process? What will I like and not like about the experience? Am I going to be strong enough? Is my baby going to be okay? Will I know how to protect her? Will I know what I want in the moment?" If you don't have a lot of questions running through your mind, you can instead ask yourself "How do I *want* to feel? What do I *want* to love about the birth process?" You don't need to have complete answers. Just start identifying and clarifying for yourself what you know about what you want.

A suggestion is to grab a blank sheet of paper or journal and write all the thoughts that come to mind as you ask yourself the questions that are top-most on your mind. For example if one of your questions is: "How long will delivery take?" you might write: "I don't want my delivery to last more than x number of hours. I want to be able to acknowledge when I move from one phase of labor to another. I'd like to be at home as much as possible. I'll need music to calm me." and so forth. Obviously each person's questions, responses, and desires could vary greatly.

When writing, don't edit yourself. Let the thoughts pop into your mind and capture your stream of consciousness. You'll begin to see what you know you want for your childbirth experience and what you're not sure about.

Check In. What do you clearly know you want for your delivery?

As Morgan considered the birth process, she felt the most enjoyable part would be the intimacy with her husband. She kept imagining what a powerful bonding experience it was going to be bringing a baby into the world together. As the images became more and more clear in her head, she realized that she wanted – as much as she could – to minimize the number of people in the room experiencing this with them. She wanted delivery to feel as intimate as possible and didn't want others talking with them or engaging with them more than was necessary. Morgan planned to give birth in a hospital. That was the "place" choice that felt most safe and sensible to her. Next, she decided to not go with the teaching hospital near her house that had an excellent reputation, but meant additional people present and the possibility of teaching going on during her delivery. Morgan felt empowered by her choice, which made it easy to respond when others questioned why she wasn't delivering at the hospital that was just down the street.

Erica's inquiry about her ideal birth experience took a different focus. Erica knew she wanted to feel proud about what she would accomplish during the delivery and she wanted to feel connected – connected with her baby, her body, and the process. To achieve that, she realized she wanted her delivery to be as "intervention-free" as possible. That realization made some of her birth-related decisions very clear. She found a midwife who was known for her "let's have things unfold naturally" approach, and she decided to not take any drugs during the process. Erica's intervention-free experience began shaping up in her mind and in her reality.

It's useful to be clear – at a high level – about what we want for our birth process. As Morgan and Erica both experienced, when we get clearer and clearer about what we'd ideally want, then we begin to notice more concretely what seems to be moving in that direction or not. We begin to see actions we could take to help ensure that we get what we want. Morgan was able to make a hospital choice about which she felt very peaceful and grounded. Erica knew the type of care provider with whom she wanted to work and the types of conversations she wanted to have with her midwife. Knowing what we want helps us move towards it, mentally, emotionally, and tangibly with the actions we take.

Additionally, when we focus on what we want, we can more readily see when what we're getting is aligned with what we want. When we have a destination, it's affirming to notice all the evidence that shows us we're on the path that will get us there.

Check In. What evidence do you have that shows you you're already creating what you want for your birth experience?

## The benefit of circular thinking

Admittedly, sometimes the questions are not as straightforward or fun as the ones Morgan and Erica dealt with. Sometimes a woman might be filled with doubt. You may have questions that look more like: "How can I stop feeling *so* overwhelmed? How will my baby and I make it through? Will I do anything that I'll regret? What if I don't know where I want to deliver? Will the hospital staff think that I am weak or whiny? How can I feel calm about birth when I have no idea how it will go?"

Many women have talked with me about the doubts that swirled around in their heads about delivery. It's easy to get down on yourself that you don't know what you want or you don't know how to quiet the insecurities that keep cycling through your mind. Instead of being thoroughly frustrated with these questions, consider instead that the swirl in your mind is an extremely useful phenomenon. The "swirl" or circular thinking is when the same thought patterns keep rotating through your mind and you're not able – for a time – to let them go or do something about them and move on.

Circular thinking – although crazily annoying at times – can provide you with insightful information; it can point you to what's most important. When you notice what your mind keeps looping back to, you can identify a concern and perhaps where it is coming from. For example, if you are continually thinking about the hospital setting and who is going to be there when you give birth, that might mean that you're concerned about how the hospital staff might judge you as a woman in labor. And, that what is most important to you is to feel comfortable and confident throughout the process. Once you know that, then you can ask yourself how you can create what you want. Do you want to jokingly apologize ahead of time that you're certain there will be a "crazy lady" portion of the program? Do you want to wear a top that brings out the color in your eyes because wearing your "best" color will boost your confidence? Do you want to decide not to care about certain things? Do you have specific requests that will help improve your comfort level? You can take a look and determine where you want to focus.

Check in. What do you have circular thoughts about regarding birth?

What concerns are your circular thoughts pointing to?

What can you do to alleviate your concerns?

As you continually uncover what's important to you, determine what you want, and take the actions that you believe are most likely to get you there, your swirly thoughts and unanswered questions will likely start to dissipate. However, there may be some that are leftover or continue to linger. What do you do with these?

## The process of discovering what you want

How do we gently accept our persistent uncertainties? This will look different for each of us. One thing to remember is that not knowing what you want for aspects of your delivery process is common and normal. You don't need to beat yourself up if you're uncertain about what you want. Even though billions of women have given birth and there's a lot we know about the process, you don't know how your particular experience will unfold or about how it will work best for *you.*

Just know that your questions keep you motivated and tuned in, and that's a good thing. Your ongoing considerations let you know what your intuition is telling you to take a closer look at. Getting clear about what you want is a process.

Bridget learned that sometimes it can take a while to discover what you want. She had decided she wanted to experience the birth of her son without an epidural. She felt certain about the decision, or so she thought. Even though she told her midwife that was her choice, doubts kept coming up for her. Second guessing the choice freaked her out for a time, and she felt really down on herself that she wasn't 100 percent certain about something to which she had thought she was passionately committed.

As she continued to reflect, she had the insight that she had made the right choice, but maybe there was something to tweak about it. Maybe she needed some way to prepare for this choice or an "out clause" for certain circumstances. This got her excited and into an exploratory mode. She researched breathing techniques, took some classes, and talked to other women. Still, her doubts didn't diminish. So she kept looking. Eventually, she learned about a unique method of relaxed, natural childbirth education that's enhanced by self-hypnosis techniques. She knew she'd found an approach that made her feel more confident and grounded in her overall choices. Bridget then stopped beating herself up about having unease about her choice and moved into fully trusting herself. She was proud she had kept looking until the swirling uncertainties were quieted.

Bridget's story points to the importance of exploring. There may not be anything to change; there may be a small tweak to be made. It may just be a process of acknowledging and understanding where your uncertainties are coming from. You can do this in many ways: talk to others, talk to a therapist or coach, journal, take a walk, etc.

You always have the opportunity to thoughtfully choose what you want for your birth experience, just as you always have the opportunity to choose what you want for your pregnancy experience. Set aside what you think you *should* choose. Look at what you've seen work well for others and consider your strengths and preferences and ask yourself if the same will work well for you. Why or why not? You don't have to answer every possible question out there. You can notice which aspects of the experience are most important to you and simply consider those. Identify, simply what you most like to see unfold for yourself and your baby.

## Using your data to make your choice

You make your choices as best you can at any given moment with the data you have. There is one kind of "data:" information about the care providers and birthing center locations in your area, breathing techniques and other birthing approaches, what you know is possible from what you've read and heard from others, how the body and the process works, statistics, and other types of researchable facts. There is also another type of data that is equally important and valid: your thoughts, feelings, and reactions to what you've read, heard, witnessed, and/or experienced. In fact, these latter pieces of data, at times, may be more important. You're never going to have *all* the facts and information, and how you think and feel about the information you have is likely to be quite telling.

Trust yourself. Do what you can to understand your true feelings and opinions and move forward. Make the best decisions that you can regarding your delivery and believe you're choosing what will work best for you. This is much easier said than done, at times, I realize. It can be easy to worry that you don't have all the information that you should or that you're making decisions about something you don't understand very well. Yet, getting worked up and worried about a circumstance you can't change doesn't serve a purpose. It doesn't help you. Instead, you want to trust: trust that you have the information you need to make the best decision for you, trust that you've processed what you need to in order to understand your own preferences, trust that you've made the best choice, trust that there's a reason you made this choice. This is a way to truly empower yourself.

Check in. What choices have you made (even if only in your own mind) about your birth process that you trust?




Why do you trust these choices?

## When we receive new data

What if we get a new piece of information that causes us to doubt a decision we've made about our upcoming delivery? What if something starts nagging at us and we're not sure we've made the right choice?

These are great questions. You want to trust yourself, especially when your intuition tells you *not* to trust a decision any longer.

You make choices and create what you want based on the data that you have in that moment. Then, as you are moving forward, taking actions, being committed to a certain course of action, you generate more data. It may be information that delights or raises concerns as you, for example, pursue delivering at a certain birthing center or talk with your care provider about a birth plan or ask your mommy friends more pointed questions. Additional information may make your decision resonate more deeply for you and feel better and better; or it may create a sense that something feels "off" or not right. In essence, layers of data build up over time and with each layer, you have the opportunity to reinforce or alter your choices. Following this cycle, you can fully trust a choice you make until your intuition and your "data" tells you it's time to make a different choice or a course-correction.

As Debi, who we met in the *Choosing Your Care and Support* chapter, sought out information about having an unassisted home birth, she felt more and more secure in her choice. The more she read about women's accounts of their home births, the more she felt like they were describing *her* experience. When people in her life expressed concerns and fear on her behalf, she was grounded enough in her choice that she didn't feel the need to take on those concerns for herself. She felt she had found her path and all the new data she received – even when it wasn't in "agreement" with her choice – continued to confirm that for her.

Ellen had a different experience. Ellen lived in Canada where it is common to have frequent in-home visits from your midwives throughout your pregnancy. This setup had sounded fabulous, easy, and luxurious to Ellen. She was really looking forward to experiencing that level of care. However, when the midwives started coming over regularly and initiating different conversations about her pregnancy and upcoming birth, she found herself annoyed. She kept trying to dismiss her feelings, thinking, "Who wouldn't want attentive, come-to-your-house care?" It was so convenient and personalized. Yet Ellen realized it was not for her. It surprised her to discover that it felt like too much.

Ellen was proud of herself for admitting that she didn't want what she, and so many others, would assume was a good thing. She knew it was great care, just not for her. She made changes to create an arrangement that felt more aligned with her true desires.

It's an interesting balance to strike as you make choices: trust you've got the data you need to make your choice, *and* allow new data to shift your choices, when and if that's appropriate.

Check in. Where are you receiving new data (information as well as your own thoughts and feelings) that is confirming your choice?

Where are you receiving new data that might lead you to make a different choice about your delivery?

## Acknowledge your decision-making abilities

Because your choices may evolve and change over time, it's great to acknowledge your decision-making abilities along the way. Acknowledge yourself for times you've made choices easily and gracefully. Acknowledge yourself for staying in the inquiry and exploring possibilities. Acknowledge yourself for struggling and feeling uncertain, knowing that you'll eventually find your way. Pat yourself on the back for everything you're doing well as you make decisions regarding this significant event in your life.

This is important because there will be times when you need to remember how far you've come and all the milestones you've achieved on your motherhood journey.

When Christine got pregnant she instantly knew where she wanted to give birth. A number of her friends recently had babies at one of the local hospitals, and Christine really liked how the facility looked and felt. It was welcoming and not at all coldly clinical. She could imagine herself laboring there and holding her baby in one of the beds. The choice resonated in her core. What she wasn't certain about was whether she wanted to have a birthing tub in her room or not. Some of her friends had used one and some hadn't. Those that had, loved the experience of being in the tub and talked about how relaxing it was and how it took your mind off the pain.

Christine just didn't know. Sometimes she felt she could imagine herself laboring in a tub. At other times she couldn't conjure up the visual. She struggled with what this meant. Did it mean that the tub wasn't for her? Did it simply mean that this was new and somewhat unfamiliar to her, so of course she couldn't fully imagine what it would be like? At times it sounded delightful to be buoyant with her baby in the water. And, at other times, she couldn't get past the logistics of what she'd be wearing, how she'd be all wet afterwards, and how she'd get in and out of the tub. She felt stuck and insecure about not fully knowing her own wishes.

After struggling for some time, one of her friends gently reminded her about how strong Christine's convictions were about many aspects of her delivery. She was simply undecided about this one. And, she had time. She could wait until she was in labor to decide. Christine took a step back and acknowledged what she had accomplished. She had made all the decisions that she had to at this point, and felt great about them all. As she reflected, she actually felt certain that the decision about the tub would be okay either way. That belief reassured her. Christine could've let her indecision unravel her. Instead, she focused on her ability to make good decisions for herself and trusted that she'd continue to do that.

Check In. What can you acknowledge and appreciate about your birth-related decision making?

In addition to acknowledging your decision-making abilities along the way, it's also important to validate your choices after the fact. When you are clear on *what* the choice was, *how* you made it, and *why* you made it, it will help guide you when a new set of circumstances comes along.

After giving birth to her son, Julie reflected on the decisions she made throughout the delivery process. She had gone into the process thinking that she wanted a natural, vaginal birth, and during the actual birth process she decided to get an epidural and add Pitocin (a synthetic form of the naturally occurring hormone, oxytocin, intended to induce and mimic normal labor). She wanted to fully sort out those choices in her mind so she wouldn't have any lingering questions.

When she had been pregnant and contemplating a drug-free delivery, her perspective had been, "Why not?" She was a strong, healthy woman. She could do it. Yet after pushing for quite some time, her baby was not moving past a certain point. Her doctor began talking about adding Pitocin and starting an epidural. Given what Julie knew about her current situation and what she had researched about the effects and possible side effects of these interventions, moving forward with the drugs made sense to her. So, she agreed. She wanted to get her baby past this portion of the birth canal.

The process immediately moved along. Julie felt she was working plenty hard pushing her baby the rest of the way, and no further intervention took place.

After reflecting on what happened and retracing her thought processes, Julie was able to validate her choices. Her approach of knowing her options and feeling educated about the possibilities during labor was important and empowering. She was glad she understood the reasons for the options presented and that she had mentally prepared herself for unexpected changes. She could look back and feel at peace with what she had decided.

It might be easy to think, "Well, of course, Julie could feel at peace with her decisions. Nothing too drastic happened!" So, how do you handle it when the choices you're presented with don't look appealing? And, how do you handle it when the choices feel like they have to be made too quickly?

## When choices need to be made quickly

Some women will tell you that parts of labor and delivery take *way* too long. And, there can be times when things progress rapidly. Especially when circumstances change and there are decisions to be made, it can feel as if everything is moving faster than your ability to process it all. It can seem like choices need to be made in an instant. How do you best handle it when delivery choices need to be made very quickly?

Madison experienced a few moments when it seemed like everything shifted during the birth of her second baby. She was laboring along nicely and knew she and her baby were doing a great job. She felt proud, peaceful, and like she was perfectly in sync with what was happening.

In a moment, this all changed. The monitors next to her bed started beeping and the hospital staff looked intense as they told her that her baby was "in distress." Madison never fully understood what this meant; she just felt the need to do something urgently. Her doctor mentioned forceps and Madison simply said, "Hurry." She was scared for her baby and wanted her out immediately where the pediatricians could get their hands on her and help her. The next minutes passed in a blur and before the forceps had successfully drawn her daughter out, the beeping stopped. The doctor removed the forceps and set them down. Calm returned for Madison just as quickly as it had disappeared a moment earlier. She once again felt like she and her daughter were right where they needed to be and doing great. About 10 minutes later her daughter was born without the use of forceps.

Afterwards, Madison thought about what had happened in those panicked moments, and she believed that she should not have agreed to the use of the forceps. Prior to that point, she had been feeling that her progress was great. She questioned why she totally forgot how secure she was feeling when the machines started beeping? Why didn't she ask about how the forceps worked? Why didn't she figure out what "in distress" meant before she panicked? She spent a good deal of time beating herself up.

Finally she gave herself a break. She realized that she'd never judge another woman as harshly as she was judging herself. It was quite understandable that she'd panic. Her nourishing mother drive was kicking in under perceived time pressure. She told herself it was natural to move into "act now" mode. Madison finally started being compassionate with herself and feeling more at peace with her choices.

Josie was confronted with time-pressured choices as well. Her water broke in the grocery store while she was shopping with her husband

and her toddler. They left the cart in the aisle with the groceries in it, dropped their son off at Grandma's house, and drove to the hospital straight away. She immediately was admitted and was administered an epidural. There was all this activity and then things slowed down. Josie was feeling contractions, yet they were far apart and fairly mild. They'd build up in intensity in one half hour and then back off the next. The speed-up, slow-down pattern was frustrating – mainly because she felt she wasn't fulfilling the expectations of the hospital staff that seemed to want her to progress more quickly. Overall, though Josie felt she and her baby were approaching birth in their way.

She had thoroughly convinced herself that things were moving forward "just right" when her doctor started talking about how they were approaching the 24-hour mark and recommended a Pitocin drip. Josie had not zeroed in to how much time had passed by and asked the staff to stop so she could think about the drip. The nurse started to argue, and even though Josie knew the nurse had the baby's best interests at heart, Josie didn't feel compelled to immediately comply. She asked everyone to leave so she and her husband could discuss what they wanted to do. Josie explained to her husband how she felt she and their baby were in their rhythm and how it didn't feel right to speed that up. She also questioned what was magical about the number 24? Were you fine in hour 24 and all of a sudden in grave danger hour 25? They asked the doctor to wait for 27 hours before moving forward with the Pitocin. The doctor agreed. Ultimately, Josie delivered her baby before that time.

Looking back, she was proud that she trusted herself and slowed the action down so she and her husband could talk. She hadn't been feeling any pressure internally. When the external pressure arrived, she was able to objectively observe the contrast between it and what was going on inside of herself. She hit the pause button and gave herself time to figure out what to do.

Check in. What do you know about your ability to make choices when you're under a time constraint?

What do you want to keep in mind if you need to make quick decisions during your delivery?

## Lessons learned in hindsight

It's easy to get into the pursuit of making perfect choices at every opportunity regarding an event as important as the birth of your child! In an ideal world, you'd want to be 100 percent assured that you had made *all* the correct decisions and that they would lead to having the best, most enjoyable birth experience possible. I know that's what I wanted! It's normal and natural to put big pressure on yourself to make all the absolute "best" or "right" choices. The tricky part is that sometimes the best or right decision doesn't fully reveal itself to be best or right until we're looking back in hindsight.

Debra had three very different birth experiences and sometimes found herself believing that some of her choices were wrong. She felt she should have known better and done something differently. Yet, when she took a larger picture view of the journey through her pregnancies and deliveries she could see the lessons learned – particularly after her second pregnancy – and how the different sets of data led to her different choices. She also saw the evolution of her desires and the possibility that all of her choices were "right" even though some felt better than others in the moment.

In her second pregnancy, Debra decided to work with a female obstetrician, after having worked with a male resident during her first. She made assumptions that the doctor would have a certain kind of demeanor and handle things in a calm, compassionate manner. She was surprised and understandably unnerved when the woman came into the room while she was in labor, turned on the lights, demanded that Debra lay down, and yelled at the nurse! Debra allowed these actions to take her out of the peaceful mindset she had been in. She was distracted and didn't enjoy the delivery as much as she thought she could. Debra believed that she put too much faith in this doctor simply because she was a woman. She learned how affected she was by the actions and energy of those around her. This lesson has proved invaluable to Debra as she's made other important decisions for her children such as which childcare providers and sitters to employ. She was glad to have had that experience and learn its lesson in such a profound way.

In her third birth, Debra moved to a midwifery model. She felt she needed to create an environment that supported her in every way. She didn't want to feel any need to "protect herself." She thought about the experience as completely pleasurable and empowering. And, she knew she wouldn't have had this experience if she hadn't had the previous ones. Coupling what she learned about keeping her intentions front and center and about how affected she is by others' energy, she created what felt practically ideal.

It can be much easier said than done, yet you want to remember that even though you might make different choices for subsequent birth experiences, it doesn't mean that what you did previously was wrong. It's possible that all the different choices were "right," even if you enjoyed some more than others. Look at what your past choices have enabled you to do.

Check in. What birth choices of yours have you judged as "wrong"?

How can you gently, compassionately accept these choices and not judge them as "wrong"?

You want to be gentle and compassionate with yourself regarding the choices you make. There is a huge and ever-growing variety of places where you can give birth, types of practitioners with whom you can work, approaches and techniques you can use to support your delivery. There are an infinite number of choices you might make in regards to your preparation, environment, care, interventions, etc. It can be overwhelming and the pressure to make just the right choices is enormous. Remember that you can't possibly know everything. You can't foresee how things will go. You don't know exactly how you'll think and feel during the process. You are not in control of all the variables. Our babies are going to be doing their own thing and all we can do is make the best choices given what we know about ourselves and our circumstances.

The goal is not to "do" the birth experience perfectly. The goal is to give birth to a baby. It's easy to lose sight of that as you are diligently working to make the best choices for you and your baby. Sometimes you need to be mindful of how you are defining "success."

Birth is an event you're rightfully passionate about, and of course, you want to create awesome birth memories for yourself. Yet, as with any other area of life, sometimes you need to keep your eye on the bigger picture and be prepared to go with the flow.

## Keeping your eye on the bigger picture

Now wait. Is there a contradiction here? We've learned about how women have benefited by distinguishing what they want for their delivery. And, we've seen how going with the flow could be helpful to women as they're experiencing the unknowns of childbirth. How can you do both at once?

It's about striking the appropriate balance between knowing enough about what you want so that you can prepare effectively for your delivery, and not getting so bogged down in details or attached to things going one particular way that you're unable to go with the flow in the moment.

Ann said that it worked best for her to focus primarily on her big picture wants: a healthy baby, a safe and comfortable process, and a light-hearted energy at the delivery. Nearly everything else she left to the moment, with just one exception. She invested a great deal of time and energy in creating a set of CDs of songs that would help her and energize her during the different stages of labor. The CDs were labeled and her husband and midwife knew exactly what she wanted to hear and when. This balance between big picture and small details worked well for Ann.

Sandra wanted to be cool and collected during her delivery process. She didn't want to be one of those women who screamed at her husband "I hate you. You are never touching me again!" She didn't want to be short-tempered with her doctor and the nurses. She wanted to be and look calm.

Sandra didn't tell anyone else about her desires. She admitted that this was partially because she had a bit of a temper and didn't want any comments – good natured or not – about how realistic (or unrealistic) her plan was. And, she figured all she had to do was be patient and nice, and that shouldn't be too hard. She wasn't committing to being that way for the rest of her life, it was just for a finite period of time. Plus, she really wanted great memories of the event. Those were her motivations.

The delivery process came on Sandra hard and fast. It seemed that one minute she felt her first contraction and the next the contractions were intense and coming regularly. She felt thrown off balance because the process was not at all progressing as she had imagined. She felt she couldn't keep up. That's when the anxiety and uncertainty began making her irritable. She needed help, but she didn't know what kind of help and her husband had no fumbling clue as to how to support her. She snapped at him. She knew she didn't want to, and she seemed helpless to stop herself. She was caught up in the swirl of emotion and didn't know how to get herself out.

As her labor progressed and Sandra got her rhythm, she was, at times, distractedly beating herself up for not being the nice and calm laboring woman that she had wanted to be. She realized in hindsight, that she wasn't, in some moments, fully able to appreciate the connection and flow that she, her baby, and her husband had created together. And that was actually what she desired more than being a perfectly calm person throughout the process. She had wanted to create an experience of love and connectedness with her family, and she had done that. She could revel in what she'd accomplished, instead of fixating on the idea that she hadn't been perfectly calm throughout. In fact, it was enlightening to learn that she could feel love and connection even when she was flustered and irritable.

Yes, you want to get clear about what you want because that helps you notice and take advantage of the opportunities to create your desired outcome. At the same time, you want to make sure that the process of deciding doesn't create a perfection mindset. It's not helpful to cling to the thought that "this process better unfold in exactly this way or else I'm going to be hugely disappointed (or feel like a failure, or be ashamed or some other negative emotion)." Focusing on bigger picture wants, such as Ann's desire to create a comfortable and light-hearted energy and Sandra's desire to feel love and connectedness, help keep you from developing a desperate need to have the process unfold in specific ways.

The trick is not getting "attached" to the process looking a certain way, reminding yourself that you're not fully in control, and preparing yourself to be able to accept and let go of what we can't control.

Check in. Where do you have an unhealthy attachment to things going a certain way?

How can you "unattach"?

## ❀ OKAY, LET'S BE REAL... ❀ ❀ ❀ ❀ ❀ ❀ ❀ ❀

*Just give me empathy!*

Often, we go to others for advice. There are many times when we want their ideas and resources. And, let's be real. There are also times – like when we have a birth experience full of unknowns looming in front of us – when we just want a little empathy! Nothing else. No problem-solving. No ideas. No "you can do it" or "you'll figure it out" encouragement. Just empathy. We want people to listen and tell us they understand our anxieties. That's all.

It would be nice if people, before they start giving advice, would pause and consider whether we've asked for any.

If this sounds and feels familiar, consider getting yourself some friends who will agree to "empathy only" conversations! Sometimes that is simply all we're interested in.

# Capitalizing on your strengths and personal attributes

What strengths might you be able to leverage during your delivery? What are you good at? If you know yourself to be a calm person or a person who's great at planning or a person who can act like a crazy, screaming maniac and then easily forgive yourself or a person with high pain tolerance or a person who gets it done when it's really important or a person who likes to be the center of attention or a person who can bring the funny into intense situations or a person who is very in tune with her body – capitalize on this. Find your strengths and exploit them. See how you can bring your unique abilities to the experience and create what best works for you.

Let's hear about how some women have capitalized on their strengths and focused on what they wanted, and thus had a self-affirming experience.

I talked with Julie when she was pregnant with her first child. She was worried about all that could go wrong. I asked her, "What's the worst that could happen?" She hesitated, said she didn't know and then listed some possibilities, none of which involved permanent damage for her or her yet-to-be-born son. I asked her, "If some or all of that happened, would you make it through?" Julie seemed confused, then she realized that yes, of course, she'd make it through. She had no doubt about that. She knew that whenever push came to shove, she knew what to do and was good in intense situations. It dawned on her that this trait would serve her really well during the delivery of her son. Acknowledging this boosted her confidence and greatly alleviated many of her worries.

Katie was loud and assertive. She was never afraid to voice her opinion. She was able to unapologetically let the hospital staff know when she wanted more ice chips, when she wanted to get up and walk around, and when she thought there were too many people in the room. As she told me about her birth, she clearly didn't feel sheepish about making her desires known in the moment. She was proud that she asked for what she wanted and had gotten everything she requested along the way. She figured that when you're the one in the room pushing a baby out of your vagina, you should get whatever your heart desires!

Marta had always known herself as someone who was great at listening to her body. She'd get messages from her body about when it was time to rest, eat some red meat, treat herself to a massage, etc. She loved and appreciated this trait about herself. When she was pregnant, she didn't know how her body would respond to labor and delivery. Yet, she also knew with certainty that she didn't have to prepare or worry ahead of time. She felt confident she'd just be able to tune in, in the moment, and know what her body wanted and needed. This assurance allowed Marta to feel peaceful and present during the birth of her daughter.

Vanessa had a great sense of humor and was proud of the fact that she could easily laugh at herself. She knew she wanted to bring some lightness and humor to the hospital delivery room to help keep her and her husband calm. She wanted to enjoy the experience and have it be fun.

At one point during her delivery, her son went into distress. To help alleviate the pressure on her baby, the doctor suggested that Vanessa get on all fours and allow her stomach to hang in the air. Her husband was in the bathroom when Vanessa made the move to this new position, and her feet and her butt were facing the bathroom door. Her humor kicked in when she thought about what her husband would see as he emerged. When she heard the door open, she looked back and demanded, "How's that view?" They laughed at the time and continue to laugh about it today. Vanessa was convinced her lightheartedness and humor kept her, her baby, and her husband relaxed and positive throughout the process.

Julia knew she was strong and flexible. No matter what physical challenge she decided to take on, she succeeded. She'd never given birth before, yet she had an inner knowing that she could do this. She reminded herself of the obstacles her body had overcome in the past: muscle sprains, broken bones, fatigue. She'd been able to work through them all. It was difficult at times to relate to herself as fit and able-bodied as her thighs grew and she felt out of breath after minimal exertion. Yet, she remembered how she had doubted herself in the past and how her body had always come through. Julia continued to focus on the strength and resilience she knew her body had and how proud she'd be when she held her baby in her arms.

Check In. What strengths and personal traits will you leverage during delivery?

Everyone has unique strengths. You have the opportunity to tap into what is distinctively "you" and make the journey as empowering and enjoyable as you can. Each of you is the only one who can say what that uniquely-yours experience looks and feels like.

## Preparing for something you've never done before

After identifying what they know they want for their delivery process and making concrete decisions, some women have found it amazingly helpful to generally prepare for an experience in which there are known factors and unknown factors. This might involve preparations such as meditation, visualization, or exercising to strengthen their bodies.

How do you prepare for something brand new? It's a valid question. And even if you've given birth before, you've never experienced *this* birth process. Each delivery is unique and there are always unknowns. It may seem challenging to try to prepare yourself when you're not sure what's going to come up. Yet, there are some things you can consider doing to feel prepared.

Many people proclaim the power of visualizing what you want. Georgia, for example, prepared for her child's birth by actively visualizing the experience she wanted to have. I asked her, "How can you visualize something you've never done?" For her, part of it was simply anticipating how she wanted to feel throughout the process – the specific kinds of emotions she'd most like to have – and she pictured herself feeling that way. Another thing that helped her was educating herself on anatomy. She looked at pictures of the cervix and understood what different muscle groups would be engaged during different stages of the process. With this knowledge she began to imagine what it would look and feel like as her body experienced different phases of the journey of birth.

Georgia visualized herself feeling confident and secure as she rode the waves of contractions in early labor. She saw herself on her feet moving around and swaying with pressure across her back and belly. She felt herself focusing on her breath. She created a picture in her mind of herself giving birth to her beautifully healthy baby.

She acknowledged that she hadn't been able to fully visualize precisely what would happen, yet she was confident that preparing her mind and body for delivery was highly valuable for her. Through her visualizations, she created a practice of allowing concerns to appear and then releasing what she didn't want to focus on. And, she strengthened her ability to focus on what she truly desired.

## Preparing in the way that feels best to you

As part of her doula practice, Jill was aware of and taught a practice called kiva in which a person becomes internally focused. It's a type of practice where you are super present to the current moment – what's going on with your feelings, your vibrational energy, and your physical body. Jill knew that she wanted the ability to transition herself to an altered state of consciousness during birth, without the use of chemicals. And, she believed that she would need to practice in order to be able to do that during the birth process.

There are an infinite number of ways to practice kiva and create that sacred, internally-focused space. In fact, Jill created kiva in distinct ways in each of her pregnancies. In her first pregnancy, Jill's kiva practices were very visual. She was coloring, drawing, and creating collages with pictures, all the while intentionally pulling herself away from external sights and sounds, such as the trees blowing outside the window and the traffic going by on the street below. With practice, she achieved regular success with attaining an internal focus that she used when she gave birth. She noticed that it was a very visual experience for her. As she pulled her focus inward, she had a sort of out-of-body experience in which she could see what she and her baby were experiencing.

Jill's second pregnancy was filled with physical kiva practices, including walking and exercising and yoga. And that birth process was quite physical. It was essentially a three-hour labor process in which she went from kneeling in a lunge to full squatting position to standing in her husband's arms as her midwife caught the baby. Along the way, Jill practiced her intentional breathing like she had in yoga and aimed to mimic the peaceful, centered feeling she'd had in so many of her physical kiva practices.

In her third pregnancy, Jill practiced auditory kiva. She repeated mantras and sang songs. Jill then had music playing during the delivery to aid her in getting to a place of internal focus where she was acutely aware of the present moment. It helped her handle whatever the birth process asked of her.

She prepared for each birth in a way that felt most intuitively right for her, and let the births themselves unfold according to what felt good and appropriate.

We each get to determine the amount and type of preparation that works for us. For example, you can complete a birth plan, talk with your care provider about his/her approach and philosophies, educate your doctor or midwife on what approaches you want carried out, attend birth classes, do kegel exercises, ask other moms the questions you have, post questions online, connect online with women who've created the type of experience you're most interested in creating. The options today are ever-expanding.

It's also important to consider what you do *not* want to do to prepare for your impending birth. This might be just as important to identify as the actions you *do* want to take to prepare. It can be easy to feel like you're *supposed* to take the recommended childbirth classes or that you *should* practice visualization or meditation to holistically ready yourself. I say not if it doesn't feel like it resonates well for you. Might you want to try something new or take yourself out of your comfort zone? Certainly. Yet, you don't want to force or pressure yourself into doing something that you don't ultimately want to do.

Check in. How do you want to prepare for your birth experience?

What are activities you know you do NOT want to do to prepare?

## The power of the "present"

A few of the women's stories in this chapter have pointed to the power of "tuning inward" or staying in the present moment. Women have found this helpful in minimizing pain and/or identifying what they want and need physically and emotionally throughout the birth process. There is another pragmatic benefit. When you're in the present you are not concerned with any past-based or future-based anxieties. When you're in the present, you can assure yourself: "I am okay. I am okay in this moment. Right now, I'm doing fine. I'm experiencing this and dealing with what is going on."

When you slip out of the present and start thinking about what might be coming in the future or what you haven't enjoyed in the past, that's the time you find yourself getting wound up and concerned. During the birth of my daughter, her heart rate dropped a number of times. All of us in the room could hear this because of how I was being monitored. The first time it happened, the doctor had me roll to my side and said that because of the decreased heart rate they wanted to expedite the delivery process. As the doctor explained her suggestions, I was thinking, "Okay, things are changing. And, everything is fine right now. My baby is fine. I am fine." I told myself to pay close attention. It almost seemed as if I was holding my breath as the doctor explained why she was suggesting the use of forceps, how the forceps worked, and how I would likely tear when we used them.

I listened calmly and when the doctor was done and seemed to be waiting for my decision, I slipped out of the present moment and panicked thinking about what might happen in the future. "What if my baby's in trouble and we don't get her out in time?" I wanted to scream, "Go, go, do it, get her out!" Then, I realized that my daughter's heart rate had increased and that the staff seemed to come out of "alert" mode. I rolled back onto my back and we agreed to continue without the forceps.

I was back in the present moment, the panic was gone, and I started to feel proud. My daughter was doing what she needed to do and she increased her heart rate all on her own. And, I also knew that, if it seemed necessary, I was fully ready to use forceps or some other intervention if we needed to get my baby out of me in a hurry. This felt good. All was well in the moment and if we needed to change course, I'd be ready to do so.

After that, my daughter's heart rate would sometimes slow right after a contraction. When it did, I would tap on my stomach and talk to her, "McKenzie, come on, I need your help, bring up your heart rate." One time, after a contraction and some pushing, I was worrying about how tired I was and wondering how long it would take and if my baby and I would be able to continue doing our work to get her born. I'd left the present moment again and was getting wound up and worried. My husband snapped me back to the present when he exclaimed, "Talk to her!" I hadn't realized that her heart rate had dropped a little again. I spoke to her right away, and knew once again we were doing well and working in partnership.

It wasn't until I reflected on the experience later that I could clearly see that the times I felt confident and knew we were safe, were the moments that I was present. When I became worried or panicked, it was because I had let my thoughts swirl ahead to a future concern that hadn't yet happened. I saw the power of staying present.

Georgia proactively thought about her intentions to remain present throughout her delivery. She knew this would help her instinctively know what to do, and she wanted to fully experience the miraculous process. Her husband reminded her of her intentions during her labor when he said, "Just concentrate on this moment." And she would close her eyes and go deeper into herself. She was so in touch with what was going on, that she could sense a change in her body temperature as she prepared for a contraction. She got cold just before a contraction and warm during the contraction. She felt so present, grounded, and clear on what her needs were. Also, by focusing on herself and the present moment, she was able to let go of thinking that she had to be polite or had to act in a certain way, and she just let herself be.

Check in. What benefits can you see for staying in the present moment during your delivery?

How will you stay in the present moment?

## When we're present, we're present to the miracle

Supriya had planned a natural, vaginal delivery. When she had been in labor for about 25 hours and pushing hard for four or five hours, it clicked in her mind that she might need a cesarean. After a few moments of struggling with that idea, she felt a flow of acceptance and thought, "Okay, let's just do a c-section." She knew she was doing a 180-degree change from the whole natural delivery that she had planned. Yet, once she reconciled the choice, she didn't feel a lot of angst. It was becoming painfully clear to her that the pushing and vaginal delivery wasn't progressing the way one would want.

She didn't voice her thoughts about the c-section out loud. She was adjusting to the idea in her own head. About two hours later the hospital staff called for an emergency c-section and Supriya was ready. She agreed, and she enjoyed the experience. She described it as "neat" when they reached into her belly. She could feel the hands inside of her, and then the hands lifting her baby out. She could feel her belly and her organs sink down when they took her son out. She didn't feel any pain, yet she could feel the sensations. She took them in and enjoyed them.

As they carried her baby past her to clean him up, she saw his legs go by and thought, "He's so beautiful. Look at those legs!" When her son started crying, she thought, "Wow, what a beautiful voice!" She watched her son in the arms of his dad, and then his aunt while they sewed her up and took care of her well-being. Yet, she didn't resent the delay at all. She was grateful loved ones were there to hold her son while she wasn't available.

I was struck by just how open and how present to the miracle Supriya was, regardless of how it showed up. There were disappointing moments when she realized she wasn't going to have a natural vaginal birth, and then she saw everything that followed as really beautiful. It wasn't exactly how she had planned, but she was still there, ready and willing to enjoy the experience.

## The emotions of birth

Throughout her birth process, Supriya experienced a range of intense emotions including frustration and anxiety as she painfully worked to push her son out; on to peace as she adjusted to the idea of a c-section; then to fascination as she felt her insides being moved around; and finally to joy, pride, and love as she saw, heard, and held her baby son. It's not unusual, as you might imagine, to feel a range of emotions and intense feelings during birth. Your baby is literally coming out of you and into the world. You are expanding and altering your family in irreversible ways. This activity is ripe for some powerful emotions!

Birth is a culmination, a transition, a beginning, a process of letting go of the way things were, and a welcoming of a new person and a new way of life. The emotions you will feel are unique and probably not entirely predictable. You may have a good idea about how you react and feel when dealing with pain and discomfort. You may have visions of what it'll look and feel like to hold your newborn baby in your arms. You may be certain that anxiety, pride, love, joy, or some other emotion is going to be part of what you experience. Yet, some unexpected emotions may come up for you as well.

During the birth of her second child, her son, Amanda had a few unexpected and seemingly inappropriate emotions surface for her. When she arrived in her hospital room, seven centimeters dilated and oh so ready for anesthesiology to arrive with her epidural, she barely noticed the various people coming in and out of the room. It was only after receiving her epidural and getting settled in, that she noticed a very good looking young doctor was in the room. He was a resident who was learning and observing. Amanda said he could stay because she wanted doctors to get as much experience and exposure as they could before they were the ones in charge. She didn't want to block that process. Yet, at the same time, she was distracted by his presence and the fact that he was quite good looking. She couldn't believe it! She was chiding herself and embarrassed that she felt vanity and increased vulnerability now that the hot resident was in the room.

To acknowledge it and bring some levity to the situation, she leaned over to her husband and whispered, "Why does the resident have to be so hot? Why is my crotch the first thing he gets to see?" Her husband giggled with her, which helped ease her mind to the idea that she was feeling something inappropriate. It took a few minutes and stronger contractions for her to stop being distracted. She was glad that she let herself fully experience and acknowledge her feelings. Amanda thought it helped her set them aside more quickly to focus on the process at hand.

Maria presumed that birth would be an intense emotional experience for her. She was one for whom "happy tears" sprung to her eyes quite often during the normal course of life. She figured she would shed quite a few tears during the process of giving birth to her baby. She assumed correctly. Her heart and soul seemed to swell with love and joy at different points in the process. She let the feelings flow and let the tears flow down her face. She didn't apologize or explain. She just let herself enjoy the moments and tried to take it all in.

What she didn't expect was the way her feelings shifted as her delivery progressed. Her emotions became directed at herself. She began to feel quite proud and felt a good deal of appreciation and love for herself.

At first she thought this was inappropriate, to have such self-centered sentiments. Then she questioned why she was trying to stop the expansion of these feelings when she hadn't tried to stop the flow of tears. She confirmed for herself that she was indeed accomplishing an amazing task and had every reason to be proud of herself. Maria did her best to let her emotions in, regardless of whether they were "expected" emotions or not.

Check in. What emotions do you expect to feel during the birth process?

Which ones are you looking forward to experiencing? Which ones are you not looking forward to experiencing?

## ✤ OKAY, LET'S BE REAL... ✤ ✤ ✤ ✤ ✤ ✤ ✤ ✤

### Permission to lose it big time!

Yes, birth is a miracle. Yes, you want it to be an experience you treaure. Yes, you want to feel empowered and grounded throughout the process. Yes, you want to generate calm for yourself, your baby, and those around you. Yes, you want to look back on what you've accomplished with pride. And let's be real, you may at some time completely lose your sh*t!

If you can give yourself permission to completely lose it during the process, do so! You might save yourself a lot of remorse. There's a lot going on and a lot is being asked of you during a short, intense period of time. It's completely understandable that you might have a little – or big – freak out.

## Reasons to fully experience emotions

Many believe it's best to allow yourself to experience whatever emotions come up as best you can. One reason is because what you resist persists. Amanda recognized that she didn't want to spend the rest of her delivery trying to pretend that the hot, young resident wasn't a distraction for her. She knew it best served her to admit to herself how she was really feeling about him being there so she could move on to more important matters. When you fully experience your emotions, you can consciously name the feelings and decide to do something intentional about them: enjoy them, let go of them, make a change in the situation, etc.

Another reason to let yourself freely experience your emotions is the belief that there's a distinct purpose for them. They can provide important lessons for you. I felt highly vulnerable and anxious about being "out of control" during the delivery process of my firstborn. Yet, after giving birth, I saw the experience differently. I was convinced that experiencing those emotions and being forced to move forward in spite of them, was meant to help me be a good parent in the multitude of situations where I would have no control. We all want the best for our children, but don't have the power to make every single thing okay. Feeling the vulnerability during birth and knowing I could proceed, even when I felt fear, was a valuable lesson.

For Amanda the benefits of feeling some twinges of vanity and attraction for the resident in the room allowed her to see that she didn't want to shut down parts of who she was just because she was now a mom. She always enjoyed appreciating a good-looking man and she didn't want to stop just because she might be holding a baby in her arms. Her delivery caused her to check for other ways she might be acting like she thought she "should," rather than how she truly wanted. Amanda knew that she could reconcile, without sacrifice, the pre-parent version of herself with the mommy version of herself.

During her delivery, Maria started the process of giving herself credit for what she did as a mom. She recognized that her children were not going to realize all that she did for them. And, they didn't have to. Maria could acknowledge and feel proud of herself.

Maria was grateful that these feelings of pride and accomplishment came up for her and that she allowed them in. She started, in those moments, an affirming and nourishing practice of thanking herself for all that she did and felt and thought about as a mom.

Check in. How willing are you to fully experience the emotions of birth?

What makes you more or less willing to experience intense emotions?

## Experiencing grief

Karen was overcome by a wave of sadness during the birth of her daughter and she believed this was part of her journey of grieving the loss of her own mother. After allowing that intense sadness during her daughter's birth, Karen felt much less of the "how am I going to be a mother when I don't have a mother" concern that plagued her during her pregnancy. She was grateful she allowed herself to freely feel her grief, even though at times she was annoyed that these emotions were part of the birth experience with her daughter. She questioned, "Haven't I already done enough to process the loss of my mom? Why does it have to come up now?" Then, she'd remind herself that obviously she hadn't. So, she let the feelings in. She knew, in the end, so much angst and grief was released as a result of her willingness and ability to be with the emotions.

Grief is often an unexpected emotion that women experience during the delivery process. This is a birth, so it can feel odd, disconcerting, or at least a bit startling to experience what is more commonly associated with death.

Yet, there are aspects of the transition of birth to grieve. There are things that you lose or things that will no longer be the same – can't be the same – after you add a child to your family. If it's your first child, your kid-less days are over. And it may sound superficial or selfish to say it (and I know as a mother of two, well worth it to give it up), yet there are things that go away: the ability to make plans at the last minute, the ability to put yourself first all the time, the freedom of not having to worry about what to feed him or whether she's getting enough sleep, the money that could be spent on fixing up the house rather than on diapers. You have another person in your life that you love with your whole heart and with that love comes responsibility and – dare I say – with burdens.

It can feel like you're giving up part of your former self as you take on this new identity of mom to your newborn baby. People will know you and relate to you in new ways. They may no longer see you as the "three margarita Saturday night" girl or as the career-driven woman or as the triathlete doing five big events a season. You may very well still be all of those things. Yet, your new mommy role will impact all areas of your life, either in how you act or how you and/or others think about your abilities to do things in the same way. Some women experience grief or other emotions about losing the life or persona they once had.

I share this not because I want grief to be an over-riding aspect of your birth experience or because I think it should be. Instead, it's one of those things that isn't often talked about. We assume birth should be only a happy, joyful place, and sometimes there are other emotions involved. I don't want you to feel alone or "wrong" if you experience something other than blissed out joy. Seemingly "negative" emotions may bubble up and it doesn't have to make the birth any less miraculous. It doesn't mean that you're not a good mother or not selfless enough if you grieve the loss of your freedom, your endless Saturday nights, your sleep, or some other aspect of your former life.

Check In. What, if anything, might you possibly grieve during the transition of birth?

# Experiencing the miracle

There's a lot that goes on throughout the delivery process that can distract us from the miracle that is taking place. It's miraculous that you are bringing a being into the world that was conceived by you and grew and developed – in millions of intricate ways – inside of you. You are altering your family and your life in inexpressible ways. You are giving birth to another. It's an amazing, miraculous happening.

You have the opportunity to find the aspects of birth that fascinate you. You can identify them ahead of time or be on the "lookout" for them as you experience the journey of birth. You may have to be intentional about this because, again, so much happens logistically during birth that can take you away from fully experiencing the miracle of the process.

Amelia loved the sensation of her daughter being born. She had an epidural so she didn't feel everything, yet she wasn't so numb that she couldn't feel the pressure and stretching. She could feel the pressure as her daughter's head and shoulders made their way out. And, it astonished her to watch her stomach going down as her baby was coming out. As the doctor lifted her daughter up and turned the baby towards her, her stomach shrunk and moved out of her view and she saw the purplish umbilical cord wrapped around her baby. It was an unforgettable sight. Amelia treasured the moments when she took in all those happenings. She thought, "Look at what we're doing! This is amazing!"

When I asked Molly about what was miraculous about her birth experience, she paused and then said what impressed her the most was that the moment her daughter was born, a family was created. Yes,

Molly was previously part of a family. Her husband had always been part of a family. Yet, when their daughter was born, they together officially created a new family – a three-person immediate family that hadn't previously existed.

In that moment, to Molly, there was a new way to relate to what she and her husband were creating. They were now the elders in their family! Molly felt the joy and pride as she was present to the shift taking place.

Carrie had waited for so long to see her babies. During her c-section, as she got her first looks at her twin son and daughter, she was overcome by joy and love and relief. It had been a long 4-year journey to this moment. She was so delighted to be on *this* side of the conception process that had involved praying, hoping, in vitro, doctor visits, disappointment, and finally success. Carrie looked at their little faces and she recognized them as her babies. She was so in love with her kids and more in love with her husband. Carrie was a mom. Her miracle was here.

Alison described her labor as very painful. As she tuned in with herself to deal with the pain, she realized that she was "hearing" clear suggestions from herself to stand this way or to labor on top of a yoga ball for a while, and so forth. It was simultaneously assuring and bizarre to her. On the one hand she had no idea what she was doing. And, on the other hand, she was receiving instinctual instructions. It was astonishing and exciting to Alison to feel like she was receiving the knowledge and experience of all the mothers who had done this before her. She felt connected to the universal community of moms, and she experienced a confidence and trust in herself stronger than any she'd ever felt before. To Alison, it was nothing short of a miracle to profoundly learn to trust herself.

Near the end of all three of her pregnancies, each of Christie's babies was in the breech position. With the birth of her first and second, Christie experienced c-sections. For her third birth experience, Christie was planning and hoping to have a vaginal birth. She'd received information, encouragement, and confidence about her ability to do so through the International Cesarean Awareness Network (ICAN).

As Christie progressed with the delivery process of her third breech baby, she was aware of how much of a hurdle and how much of a privilege it was for her to simply be a woman in labor as the process progressed. She felt honored, nervous, and confident almost all at the same time. She was able to "be with" her fears, to let them in and experience them, even as she was cognizant to not take this experience for granted. Many women with breech babies don't get to the phases of labor that she was reaching. It was a special experience.

When Christie felt they had nearly reached the moment in which she'd give birth, she asked her husband to go get a mirror. When he held it down for her, Christie could see her baby's foot coming! She described it as the most exciting moment in her entire life. She was about to give birth, to push her baby out! She'd previously assumed this would never be possible for her. Now what was previously impossible was a reality.

I love to hear women share about their birth stories, especially when a woman has a very different experience from one delivery to the next. And I love it when we are able to talk about each with such love and honor and pride, and appreciate the various aspects of each experience. No matter the circumstances, it is quite an accomplishment. We bring people – little spirits – into the world. We create. We create life. It's amazing. I'd love for us all to be present to that. And for each of you to discover and enjoy what, for you, is most miraculous about the process.

Check In. What do you know you'll enjoy about your birth process?

## ❋ Experiencing the miracle of birth ❋ ❋ ❋ ❋ ❋

You spend many months looking towards your ultimate goal: the birth of your baby. It can feel like you've only got one shot at it and had better get it "right." The birth of your baby is a miracle and may bring with it a whole range of experiences and emotions. You have the opportunity to answer for yourself: How do I create the birth experience I want, bringing my unique talents and perspectives, while knowing that I do not have complete control?

* Determining what you want for the birth of your baby helps you prepare yourself physically and emotionally for your unique birth process.

* If you're uncertain about what you want for an aspect of the process, keep exploring. Remember that you want to feel confident and empowered about your choice and it's okay to take the time you need in order to feel that way.

* Fully trust your choices and how you made your choices until your intuition tells you not to trust anymore.

* Just because you're making a different choice now than you have previously, it doesn't mean that your prior choices were "wrong" or "bad."

* You want to set yourself up as best you can for the process you most desire, while making sure you're not going to feel badly if you don't experience *exactly* what you most desire.

* You can leverage your strengths and unique traits during birth.

* There are many ways you can prepare for birth, even when you don't fully know what the experience will be like. And, you only want to engage in preparation activities that feel good and inspiring to you.

* Staying in the present moment keeps you away from future-based worries that haven't happened and helps you recognize the miracle taking place.

* A range of intense emotions may come up for you during birth. It may be beneficial – in ways you can't currently imagine – to allow yourself to fully and freely experience these emotions.

* No matter the specific circumstances, every birth is a miracle.

Check In. What are the approaches and mindsets that will enable you to most freely and fully experience the miracle of birth?

# Conclusion

I hope you found the stories and concepts shared in this book to be useful. My intent was to provide ideas and inspiration by sharing the experiences of the women who've gone before you. And, I know, at the end of the day, it's up to you. It's up to you to determine the choices that are best aligned with how you want to be as a pregnant person. It's up to you to find the mindsets that will most empower you. It's up to you to discover the ways to love the pregnant you. And, I hope you do.

I wish you a safe, blessed, and enjoyable pregnancy journey.

If you'd like to share about the successes you've had during your pregnancy, I'd love to hear from you. Others would love to hear from you!

How have you loved the pregnant you? Share on the Loving the Pregnant You blog site at http://lovingthepregnantyou.com/2011/how-did-you-love-the-pregnant-you/.

*(Or go to www.lovingthepregnantyou.com, click on "Blog," scroll down and search for "How did you love the pregnant you" and the "How did you*

*love the pregnant you?" will be one of the blog entries that appears in your search results.)*

Thank you. By intentionally creating a pregnancy and childbirth that works well for you, it makes a difference in the world. It makes a difference for you and your immediate family as you're discovering how to best enjoy the experience. And I also believe it continues to evolve the societal conversation around pregnancy in a positive way. When you insist upon doing pregnancy your unique way, you are letting people know that there are more and more choices out there and that it's okay to always be considering what's going to work best for you uniquely. You are letting people know that you want to be supported in your choices. You are letting future mothers know that they are empowered.

I'd encourage you to share about your pregnancy and childbirth experiences. Let others know about what worked for you. Not because other people should do exactly what you did. Yet, instead, to let others know that they, too, can discover what best resonates for them.

There are so many aspects of the pregnancy and childbirth experience that are not shared in everyday, mainstream conversations – such as highly hormonal moments, disappointment when our bodies don't do what we want or expect, mucus plugs, delivering the afterbirth, pee control (or lack thereof), insecurities about becoming a mom, etc. We could name many more pregnancy-related phenomena that are not readily discussed, I'm sure. And, I think the more we demystify the process and let others know what really happens, the greater the gift we give to future moms.

When we let others know about the weird, the disconcerting, the gross, and the concerning; then they don't feel weird or as concerned when something similar happens to them. Sharing the whole of the experience is vulnerable and embarrassing at times, certainly. And, I know the times I've stepped out of my comfort zone to share, I've learned that I'm not alone. Knowing that you are not alone and, at the same time, creating your own unique experience is a powerful way to approach pregnancy.

Continue to grant yourself permission to make the choices that you know will serve you best, to participate in the activities that will fuel you the most, to approach the process as you best see fit, and to be gentle and compassionate with yourself along the way. It's easy to feel judged by others and to judge yourself. Persistently strip away what you feel you "should" do to find what you truly want to do. When you are able to do that, you'll experience empowerment and peace. When you discover what you want and allow yourself to fully pursue it, you will actually be free of judgment – free from judging yourself, others, or the situation. Being totally at peace with your choices, enables you to more easily honor others' choices.

I love that vision for the world: a world where we simply empower ourselves to discover what works best for us, and in the process, we're able to eliminate judgment. When we hear an approach that is contrary to our preferred approach, instead of assessing why the choice is a "bad" one, we work to understand why the choice resonates for the other person. We embrace the idea that each person can find her unique way and that there aren't any "wrong" ways. We empower each woman to be pregnant in her unique way, so she can fully love and honor herself as she's expecting.

Thank you for being on this journey with me.

Love and blessings to you,
Amy